Drug Directory *with* Dosages *and* Indications

The other CBS books by Dr UN Panda

- *Back Pain*
- *Healthy Living: An Approach to Positive Health*
- *Doctor's Ready References*
- *Practical Prescriber with Differential Diagnosis*
- *Textbook of Medicine*
- *An Introduction to Geriatrics*

Drug Directory *with* Dosages *and* Indications

UN Panda MD
Ex-Associate Professor
Department of Medicine
Kalinga Institute of Medical Sciences
Bhubaneswar
Odisha

Pratyasha Padhi MD
Bhubaneswar
Odisha

CBSPD

CBS Publishers & Distributors Pvt Ltd

New Delhi • Bengaluru • Chennai • Kochi • Kolkata • Lucknow • Mumbai
Hyderabad • Jharkhand • Nagpur • Patna • Pune • Uttarakhand

Disclaimer

Science and technology are constantly changing fields. New research and experience broaden the scope of information and knowledge. The authors have tried their best in giving information available to him while preparing the material for this book. Although all efforts have been made to ensure optimum accuracy of the material, yet it is quite possible some errors might have been left uncorrected. The publisher, the printer and the authors will not be held responsible for any inadvertent errors or inaccuracies.

Drug Directory *with* **Dosages** *and* **Indications**

ISBN: 978-93-5466-741-1

First Edition: 2024

Published by **Satish Kumar Jain** and produced by **Varun Jain** for

CBS Publishers & Distributors Pvt Ltd

4819/XI Prahlad Street, 24 Ansari Road, Daryaganj, New Delhi 110 002, India
Ph: 011-23289259, 23266861 Website: www.cbspd.com; e-mail: delhi@cbspd.com

Corporate Office: 204 FIE, Industrial Area, Patparganj, Delhi 110 092, India
Ph: 011-49344934 Fax: 011-49344935 e-mail: publishing@cbspd.com; publicity@cbspd.com

Branches

- **Bengaluru:** Seema House 2975, 17th Cross, K.R. Road, Banasankari 2nd Stage, Bengaluru 560 070, Karnataka, India
  Ph: +91-80-26771678/79 Fax: +91-80-26771680 e-mail: bangalore@cbspd.com
- **Chennai:** 7, Subbaraya Street, Shenoy Nagar, Chennai 600 030, Tamil Nadu, India
  Ph: +91-44-26680620, 26681266 Fax: +91-44-42032115 e-mail: chennai@cbspd.com
- **Kochi:** 42/1325, 1326, Power House Road, Opposite KSEB, Power House, Ernakulum 682018, Kochi, Kerala, India
  Ph: +91-484-4059061–65 Fax: +91-484-4059065 e-mail: kochi@cbspd.com
- **Kolkata:** 147, Hind Ceramics Compound, 1st Floor, Nilgunj Road, Belghoria, Kolkata 700056, West Bengal, India
  Ph: +91-33-25330055/56 e-mail: kolkata@cbspd.com
- **Lucknow:** Basement, Khushuma Complex, 7 Meerabai Marg (behind Jawahar Bhawan), Lucknow 226001, UP, India
  Ph: +91-522-4000032 e-mail: tiwari.lucknow@cbspd.com
- **Mumbai:** PWD Shed, Gala No. 25/26, Ramchandra Bhatt Marg, Next JJ Hospital, Gate No. 2, Opp. Union Bank of India, Noorbaug, Mumbai 400009, Maharashtra, India
  Ph: +91-22-66661880/89 e-mail: mumbai@cbspd.com

Representatives

- **Hyderabad** 0-9885175004
- **Patna** 0-9334159340
- **Jharkhand** 0-9811541605
- **Pune** 0-9664372571
- **Nagpur** 0-8692091830
- **Uttarakhand** 0-9716462459

Printed at: Sri Prints and Sales, Delhi, India

to

Late Padamsree Dr LC Gupta, MD

who initiated me to the

Art of Writing

Preface

Drug Directory with Dosages and Indications is a small but handy and useful work depicting marketed drugs, their dosages and therapeutic indications.

It is very useful for students of medicine, pharmacy and nursing, medical practitioners and allied health science professionals.

All suggestions and comments for improvement are cordially welcome. My sincere gratitude to Mr YN Arjuna and his staff at CBS Publishers & Distributors in bringing out this book.

UN Panda

Pratyasha Padhi

Contents

Part II: Drugs of Last Decade

Part III: Glimpses from Pharmacology

Part I

Pharmaceutical Drugs

A

Abacavir	Anti HIV agent, 300 mg, BID
Abaloparatide	Synthetic analog of PTH, used in osteoporosis, under evaluation
Abarelix	Long-acting GNRH antagonist for cancer prostate
Abemaciclib	CDK 4/6 inhibitor for breast cancer like palbociclib, ribociclib
Abciximab	GP IIb/IIIA antagonist, used in acute coronary syndrome; 0.25 mg/kg bolus then infusion, up to 10 μg/kg 12 hourly.
Abatacept	Soluble fusion protein (CTLA–4 and IgG) used in rheumatoid arthritis, 500 mg IV at 0, 2, 4 weeks, then every 4 weeks.
Abiraterone	CYP17 inhibitor, antiandrogen for prostate cancer, 250 mg × 4 tab daily.
Acamprosate	Used in alcoholism, up to 2 g/day in 3 divided doses
Acebutolol	Antiarrhythmic agent, 200–400 mg PO BID
Acetaminophen	Paracetamol or analgesic, antipyretic; Dose 500 mg–1 g TID
Acetazolamide	Diuretic for intracranial hypertension, idiopathic intracranial hypertension, angle closure glaucoma, seizure, hyperkalemic periodic palsy: Dose—250–375 mg PO, OD
Acetylcystine	For cystitis, paracetamol poisoning; 140 mg/kg PO, then 70 mg/kg 4 hourly
Acetylsalicylic acid	Analgesic, 650 mg, PO QID (cyclooxygenase inhibitor)
Acalabrutinib	2nd generation BTK inhibitor for CLL

Acitretin	Retinoid for use orally in psoriasis; 10–25 mg PO daily
Aclidinium	LAMA for bronchial asthma
Acotiamide	Acetycholine release enhancer, used in functional dyspepsia
Actinomycin D	Antineoplastic agent, for gestational trophoblastic tumor, 0.04 mg/kg IV
Adrenaline	Sympathomimetic, 0.04 mg SC/IV in anaphylaxis
Acyclovir	Antiviral for HSV, HZV; oral 400–800 mg TID, IV 10–20 mg/kg daily
Adalimumab	TNF alfa inhibitor, for rehmatoid arthritis, 40 mg every other week
Adefovir	Antiviral for HBV, 1.0 mg/day PO
Adenosine	Antiarrhythmic agent 6–12 mg IV bolus
Afatinib	Tyrosine kinase inhibitor for lung cancer
Adapalene	1% gel for acne
Aflibercept	VEGF antagonist for macular degeneration
Albendazole	Anthelmintic for ascariasis, capillariasis, cutaneous larva migrans [400 mg tab once], tapeworm for 3 days, also for cysticercosis, echinococcosis, hook worm, trichuriasis, filariasis, microsporidiasis
Albiglutide	Long acting GLP receptor agonist for diabetes, 30 mg weekly SC
Aldesleukin (IL_2)	6 lac units/kg IV every 8 hours for 14 doses
Albuterol	β2 agonist for acute management of hyperkalemia
Alectinib	Tyrosine kinase inhibitor for lung cancer
Alemtuzumab	Immunosuppressant for multiple sclerosis, myeloid dysplasia, hypereosinophilic syndrome Dose – 30 mg SC three times per week

Alendronate	Bisphosphonate for osteoporosis, 40 mg PO daily
Alirocumab	PCSK9 inhibitor for hyperlipidemia; 150 mg 2 weekly
Aliskiren	Renin inhibitor for hypertension and diabetic nephropathy; 150–300 mg OD
Alogliptin	DPP4 inhibitor for diabetes mellitus; 50 mg daily
Allopurinol	For gout, hyperuricemic nephropathy; 300–900 mg PO daily
Almotriptan	For migraine, selective 5HT receptor agonist; 12.5 mg; maximum 25 mg daily
Alosetron	Serotonin receptor modulator for IBS like cilansetron, tropisetron
Alprazolam	Benzodiazepine for anxiety, panic disorder 0.5–2 mg PO
Alosetron	For diarrhea dominant IBS; 0.5 –1 mg BID PO
Alprostadil	Intracavernosal injection to facilitate penile erection
Alteplase (rtPA)	Recombinant tPA for coronary, pulmonary and carotid thrombolysis; 100 mg IV st
Altretanine	Alkylating agent for ovarian cancer, 260 $mg/m^2/day$ PO
Alvimopan	Peripherally acting opioid antagonist
Amantadine	Antiviral agent, for influenza, 100 mg BID; also for parkinsonism, 100–400 mg daily
Anandamide	Endogenous cannabinoid
Andaxanent	Alfa antifactor Xa for excess epixaban, dabigatran
Ambrisentan	Endothelin receptor antagonist for pulmonary hypertension
Amikacin	Aminoglycoside 15–30 mg/kg day/ (mxm—1 g), for gram–negative organism and tuberculosis

Amiloride	K^+ retaining diuretic, 5–10 mg OD/BID
Aminophyllin	Bronchodilator
Aminosidine (Paromomycin)	Aminoglycoside given orally for amoebiasis, giardiasis, cutaneous leishmaniasis
Amiodarone	Antiarrhythmic agent for tachyarrhythmia, 5 mg/min IVst, then 1 mg/min
Amitriptyline	For migraine, chronic pain, tension headache; 150 mg/day
Amithiozone	(thiacetazone) bacteriostatic antitubercular drug
Amantadine	Antiviral, used for influenza prophylaxis, SSRI related sexual dysfunction
Amineptine	Antidipressant, 100 mg BID
Amenamevir	Antiviral for HSV_1, HSV_2, inhibits helicase primase heterotrimeric complex
Amifostin	910 mg/m^2 IV before ifosfamide, endoxon; prevention of chemo toxicity
Amiloride	Diuretic used in ascites, hypertension, nephrogenic diabetes insipidus, Liddle syndrome; 5–10 mg daily
Aminoglute-thimide	Adrenal steroid inhibitor, 1000 mg PO daily
Amlodipine	Calcium channel blocker, antihypertensive, 5–10 mg OD
Amodiaquine	Antimalarial, prevents haemozoin formation, 600 mg single dose
Amoxapine	Antidepressant, blocks norepinephrine and serotonin reuptake; 100 mg BID/TID
Amoxicillin	Aminopenicillin, effective against gram–positive and some gram–negative organisms, anthrax, actinomycosis, leptospira, lyme disease, 250–600 mg TID
Amphetamine	CNS stimulant often abused, can cause cardiomyopathy, vasculitis, alopecia, fatigue

Amphotericin B	Antifungal antibiotic, lipid soluble form is more effective, 3–5 mg/daily; effective in deep-seated mycosis; coccidioidomycosis, mucor mycosis
Ampicillin	Aminopenicillin, effective for leptospira, HACEK organisms, clostridia Used in combination with sulbactam/ clavulanate 1 g IV TID
Amprenavir	Protease inhibitor, anti HIV; 1200 mg twice daily
Amrinone	A bipyridine, inhibits phospho diesterase to cause vasoconstriction
Amyl nitrite	Vasodilator, for angina pectoris; 0.3 ml cap for inhalation
Anagliptin	DPP4 inhibitor for diabetes mellitus
Atosiban	Oxytocin antagonist
Arbekacin	Akin to amikacin, 1–3 mg/kg/day IM/IV
Anagrelide	A quinazoline derivative used to treat essential thrombocytosis and polycythemia vera
Anakinra	Soluble IL–1 receptor antagonist used in rheumatoid arthritis; Muckle Well's syndrome, Still's disease, juvenile onset inflammatory arthropathy; 100 mg SC daily
Anastrozole	Aromatase inhibitor like letrozole, exemestane, 1 mg PO OD
Ancord	Pit viper venom extract for stroke (thrombolytic)
Anidulafungin	Azole antifungal for disseminated candidiasis, 100 mg IV daily
Antithymocyte-globulin	Anti CD_{52} monoclonal antibody used for myelodysplasia, aplastic anemia, post-transplant immunosuppression
Apalutamide	Antiandrogen used in breast cancer as adjuvant therapy

Apomorphine	For Parkinson's disease, 2–5 mg daily
Apixaban	Factor Xa inhibitor, oral anticoagulant for DVT, stroke prevention in cardiac disease (AF, valvular disease); 2.5 mg PO twice daily–10 mg BID
Apraclonidine	Antiglaucoma eye drop; 0.5% 1 drop TID
Apremilast	Phosphodiesterase 4 inhibitor for psoriasis, psoriatic arthropathy, Behcet's syndrome, orally twice daily
Aprepitant	Substance P/neurokinin-1 receptor antagonist for nausea and vomiting of chemotherapy; 125 mg on day 1, 80 mg on days 2, 3
Argatroban	Thrombin inhibitor for DVT, pulmonary embolism; IV infusion
Aripiprazole	Antipsychotic, second generation; 15 mg OD
Armodafinil	Alerting agent, improves daytime somnolence in multiple sclerosis
Arte ether	Artemisinin derivatives of plant, *artemisia annua* is used to treat malaria, their concentration in parasitized RBCs is 100 times than normal RBC. 150 mg IM daily × 3 days
Arte mether Arterolane	For PF malaria, 80 mg with 480 mg lumefantrine
Artesunate	For PF malaria; 2.4 mg/kg single dose IV
Arsenic trioxide	For promyelocytic leukemia; 0.15 mg/kg IV daily
Asacol	Enteric coated mesalamine like deizical, used to treat IBD
Ascorbic acid	Vit C for scurvy; 500–1000 mg daily
Asenapine	Second generation antipsychotic, 10–20 mg/day
Asparginase	Used for treatment of ALL; 6000–10, 000 IU/m^2 IV daily × 3

Aspirin	Analgesic–anti–inflammatory, also used for CAD prophy laxis, colorectal cancer prophylaxis, niacin associated flushing, preeclampsia, prevention of tension headache, rheumatic fever. Dose – 325 mg
Atazanavir	Anti HIV, protease inhibitor, 400 mg QID
Atenolol	Beta blocker for hypertension, adrenergic symptoms of Graves' disease, IHD Dose – 25–100 mg PO daily
Atezolizumab	PDL, blocker for NS CLC, urothelial cancer 75 mg/m^2 SC daily for 7 days
Atosiban	Oxytocin antagonist for preterm labor
Azacitidine	Anti cancer agent used in AML, myelodysplasia
Azathioprine	2–3 mg/kg, PO then 1–2 mg/kg maintenance, for rheumatoid arthritis; tissue transplant, autoimmune diseases
Aparanenone	Mineral corticoid antagonist like esaxerinone (investigational)
Atorvastatin	Used to treat hyperlipidemia, 20–80 mg daily
Atomoxetine	Used for treatment of orthostatic hypotension in combination with yohimbine
Atovaquone	Hydroxy naphthoquinone derivative, inhibits malaria parasite mitochondrial electron transport, for malaria prophylaxis and babesiosis; 750 mg SC/PO
Atropine	Parasympatholytic, used in anaesthesia premedication, snake bite, organophosphorus poisoning, AV conduction/SA node conduction block—0.6 mg IV infusion, 1% eye drop, mydriatic for uveitis, ointment
Avanafil	Phosphodiesterase inhibitor used in male erectile dysfunction, BPH; 50–100 mg PO

Avolumab	Anti PDL (1) inhibitor used for treatment of metastatic Merkel cell carcinoma
Avibactam	Combined with ceftazidime, a beta lactamase inhibitor akin to sulbactam, calvulanate, tazobactam and vaborabactam
Avobenzone	A sunscreen constituent, 3%
Axitinib	VEGF pathway inhibitor for RCC, others in this group are pazopanib, lenvatinib/ cabozantinib
Azathioprine	Mercaptopurine analog, inhibits hepatic purine synthesis, used in lymphoid malignancy, bullous pemphigoid, reactive arthritis, IBD, SLE, vasculitis, sarcoidosis, myasthenia gravis, multiple sclerosis
Azelaic acid	Used locally for acne vulgaris
Azelastine	Nasal vasoconstrictor useful for allergic, vasomotor rhinitis
Azlocillin	Broad spectrum penicillin effective for Proteus and Pseudomonas
Azithromycin	A macrolide antibiotic, effective for gram–positive organisms, scrub typhus, trachoma, pertusis, Mycoplasma, Legionella, gonococci, enteric fever, treponematosis, leptospirosis, babesiosis; 250–500 mg OD
Aztreonam	Monobactam effective against gram–negative organisms, structurally related to Ceftazidime; 30 mg/kg, IM/IV 8 hourly

B

Bacampacillin	200–400 mg tab, for respiratory infection, 1 tab BID
Bacitracin	Locally acting antibiotic, hampers cell wall synthesis
Baclofen	Used for dystonia, GERD, hiccup, tardive dyskinesia, in trigeminal neuralgia, 10 mg PO BID/TID
Balofloxacin	Quinolone; 100–200 mg BID
Baloxavir	Antiinfluenza agent, 40–80 mg PO daily
Balsalazide	Amino benzoyl 5 ASA used in IBD; 6.75–9 g/day
Baricitinib	Tyrosine kinase inhibitor, 4 mg daily for 14 days in COVID-19
Basilizimab	CD25 (IL-2a) receptor antibody used in graft vs host disease in bone marrow transplantation
Bapinezumab	Anti myeloid antibody like solanezumab, adocanumab, used in marrow transplantation
Bazedoxifene	For premenopausal symptoms like raloxifene
Bedaquiline	Diarylquinoline antibiotic given in MDR TB
Bazedoxifene	A SERM, marketed in combination with conjugated estrogen for treatment of postmenopausal osteoporosis (other two used for same are tamoxifen and raloxifen)
BCG	Intravesical immunotherapy for transitional cell bladder cancer
Beclomethasone	Inhaled steroid for bronchial asthma

Belatacept	Fusion protein binding to CD 80 and 86 with T cell apoptosis, used in postrenal transplant
Belimumab	Used in SLE without active renal disease, 10 mg/kg IV week 0, 2, 4
Belinostat	HDAC inhibitor for multiple myeloma
Benarotine	Topical retinoid, 1%
Benidipine	Antihypertensive, 4 and 6 mg tab OD
Benzathine-penicillin	Penicillin used in rheumatic fever prophylaxis, syphilis and endemic treponomatosis; 1.2 mU IM
Benazepril	Diuretic for hypertension; 5, 10, 20 mg OD
Bendamustine	Alkylating agent used in treatment of lymphomas and myeloma; 70–90 mg IV on day 1, 8
Benefluorex	Appetite suppressant
Benzbromarone	Uricosuric drug used in gout with nephropathy
Benserazide	Anti Parkinsonism; given with levodopa
Benznidazole	Oral nitroimidazole used in Chaga's disease; 5 mg/kg/day, 2 doses
Benzthiazide	Thiazide diuretic, 25/50 mg daily, PO
Benzonatate	Acts on cough reflex pathway, antitussive agent
Benzidamine	Oral antiseptic, mouthwash
Benzoyl peroxide	Topical agent for acne
Beractant	Phospholipid for intratracheal use in infant respiratory distress, Covid-19; 100–200 mg
Benzphetamine	Sympathomimetic anorexic agent for weight loss
Benztropine	Used in Parkinsonism
Betamethasone	Corticosteroid
Betahistine	Anti vertigo agent; 8–16 mg TID

Betaxolol	Beta blocker used in HTN. IHD; 10–20 mg OD
Bethanecol	Used in detrusor–sphincter dyssynergia, depression; 25 mg TID
Bethanidine	Anti hypertensive agent
Betrixaban	Anti coagulant for pulmonary embolism; 80 mg daily PO
Bexarotene	Retinoid, for CTCL, 75 mg PO OD
Bevacizumab	Anti VEGF used in colorectal, breast. brain, hepatic, lung, ovary and renal cancers and macular degeneration. Dose 5 mg/kg IV fortnightly
Betaxolol	0.5% eye drop for glaucoma
Bifonazole	Local antifungal
Bicalutamide	Pure androgen antagonist used in prostate cancer, 50 mg PO daily
Bictegravir	Anti HIV, 50 mg daily (in combination, only)
Biolimus	Used in drug eluting stent, other agents used for this purpose are everolimus and zotarolimus
Binatoprost	Anti glaucoma eye drop 0.03% one drop once daily
Bipenem	Broad spectrum antibiotic akin to meropenem, 1 g IV BID
Bisacodyl	Purgative, 10 mg tab, also suppository
Bisphosphonates	Used in hypercalcemia, osteoporosis, Paget's disease
Bisoprolol	Beta blocker for CHF, 1.25–10 mg OD
Bithionol	Drug that causes topical photo allergic reaction
Bismuth-subsalicylate	Used for diarrhea
Bisoprolol	Beta blocker used in coronary artery disease

Bleomycin	Antitumor antibiotic, used in ovarian, testicular malignancy; 15 units/m^2 SC/IM/IV twice weekly to total dose of 200 units/m^2
Bivaluridin	Anticoagulant used in CAD, 0.75 mg/kg IV bolus then infusion of 1.75 mg/kg/hour
Blinatumomab	CD 19 antibody used in ALL
Boceprivir	Antiviral for HCV, genotype I (Ist generation)
Bortezomib	Proteasome inhibitor for multiple myeloma, transplant rejection, amyloidosis, NHL, Waldenstrom's macroglobulinemia; 1.3 mg/m^2 IV/SC on day 1, 8, 15
Bosutinib	Tyrosine kinase inhibitor for CML
Bosentan	Endothelin receptor antagonist for pulmonary hypertension akin to tezosentan
Botulinum toxin	Used in spasticity, migraine, tics, achalasia, essential tremor, hyper hydrosis, anal fissure
Brentuximab	Brentuximab vedotin–Anti CD 20 for Hodgkin's disease, anaplastic lymphoma
Brexpiprazole	Antipsychotic agent; 1–4 mg/day
Brimonidine	Antiglaucoma eye drop 0.2%, 1 drop twice daily
Bretylium	Antiarrhythmic agent
Brivanib	First line drug for advanced hepatocellular carcinoma
Brivaracetam	Antiseizure agent; 100–200 mg BID
Bromocriptine	Oral dopamine agonist for prolactinoma, acromegaly and diabetes mellitus
Brinzolamide	Carbonic anhydrase inhibitor antiglaucoma eye drop
Bromhexine	Mucolytic, ingradient of cough expectorant
Bucindolol	Beta blocker

Buclizine	Drug for motion sickness, 25 mg tab, syrup inj. day
Budesonide	Steroid for inhalation in asthma, COPD; also nasal drop for nasal allergy
Bufadienolide	A glycoside in toad causing hyperkalemia
Bumetanide	Diuretic, used in hypertension, 0.5–5 mg daily
Bupivacaine	Local anaesthetic 2.5–5 mg for spinal anaesthesia
Buprenorphine	Used for opium withdrawal programme; 3–20 μg/hour, transdermal patch
Buserelin	LHRH agonist, SC/nasal, 1 mg, for prostate cancer
Buspirone	5 HT agonist used in anxiety, depression, SSRI related sexual dysfunction, 7.5 mg, also in nicotine withdrawal programme
Bupropion	Used for depression, smoking cessation; 250–450 mg/day
Busulfan	Anticancer agent for CML; 1.3 mg/m^2/ day PO or 4–8 mg daily
Butabarbitol	Barbiturate
Butaconazole	Antifungal for candidiasis
Butenafine	Local antifungal, 1% cream
Butoxamine	Selective β_2 blocker
Butorphanol	Opium derivative for pain management, nasal spray, 1 mg/2 mg injection
Butoform	Local soothing and anaesthetic agent, ingredient of antihemorrhoid ointment
Butamben	Local anaesthetic

C

Cabergoline	0.5 mg per week in hyperprolactinemia
Caffeine	CNS stimulant present in tea, coffee; for hypnic headache, migraine
Calcipotriene	Vitamin D analog for psoriasis, local use
Cabotegravir	Anti HIV, integrase inhibitor
Calcitonin	Hypocalcemic peptide used in osteoporosis management and Paget's disease, 100 units SC daily
Calcitriol	Vit D derivative used in hypocalcemia rickets, osteodystrophy and tetany in premature babies
Canagliflozin	$SGLT_2$ inhibitor for diabetes mellitus; 100–300 mg OD
Canakinumab	IL–1β antibody for familial Mediterranean fever
Cangrelor	P_2 Y_{12} inhibitor used in acute coronary syndrome, (platelet reversible inhibitor), 30 μg/kg bolus, then 4 μg/kg/via infusion
Candesartan	Diuretic, used in CHF, 8–32 mg OD
Capecitabine	Antimetabolite used in cancer colon, stomach and breast; 1250 mg/m^2 PO BID
Capreomycin	Cyclic peptide antibiotic used in MDR tuberculosis; 15 mg/kg/day IM
Capasaicin	Counter irritant, used as gel to treat joint pain
Capsofungin	Injectable antifungal
Captopril	ACE inhibitor used in CHF, captopril renography for diagnosis of renovascular disease; 6.25–50 mg TID
Carbacol	Choline ester, enhances bladder contraction

Carbamazepine	Antiepileptic, also used in trigeminal neuralgia, epilepsy, neuropathy; 200–300 mg TID
Carbapenem	Ertapenem, impenem, meropenem belong to this group, effective against anaerobes, gram–negative organism and MDR tuberculosis
Carbenicillin	Broad spectrum penicillin
Carbenoxolone	Glycyrrhizin derivative having anti-inflammatory action and aldosterone like activity, used in gastric ulcer
Carbidopa–levodopa	Dopa agonist used in Parkinsonism tab; 25/100, 25/250 mg
Carbidopa–levo-dopa-entacapone	Dopa agonist used in Parkinsonism 12.5/50/200 to 50/200/200 mg tab
Carbimazole	Anti thyroid, used in hyperthyroidism
Carboplatin	Antitumor agent, used in testicular cancer, lung cancer, melanoma
Carboprost	For cervical cancer; up to 1600 mg/m^2 IV in divided doses
Carnitine	Agent for cardiac health, antianginal
Carfizomib	Proteasome inhibitor, for multiple myeloma; 20–50 mg/m^2 IV
Cariprazine	Antipsychotic agents; 1.5–6 mg/day
Carisoprodol	Centrally acting muscle relaxant given PO
Carmustine (BCNU)	Alkylating agent for brain tumors, HD, NHL, MM, 200 mg/m^2 IV every 6 weeks
Carvedilol	Betablocker for CHF, 3.125–25 mg BID
Cation exchange resin	Sodium polystyrene sulfonate, used orally in hyperkalemia to promote K$^+$ loss in stool
Casirivimab	Used with imdevimab for Covid-19
Capsofungin	Antifungal for Candida, preventive therapy in neutropenia, sepsis, septic shock; 50–70 mg infusion daily

CCNU - (Carmustine)	Used to treat astrocytoma
Cefaclor	2nd generation cephalosporin for community acquired pneumonia, 500 mg PO BID/TID
Cefadroxil	500 mg BID PO
Cefamandole	2nd generation cephalosporin, for community acquired pneumonia; 2 g IV 6 hourly
Cefazolin	1st generation, against skin infection, 1–2 g IV 8 hourly
Cefdinir	3rd generation, cephalosporin, 600 mg PO daily
Cefditoren	400 mg PO BID
Carporitide	Vasodilator like ularitide (investigational)
Cefepime	Broad spectrum cephalosporin, 2 g IV TID
Cefixime	3rd generation cephalosporin, 400 mg PO BID
Cefoperazone	2 g IV BID
Cefotaxime	3rd generation cephalosporin, 2 g IV TID
Cefotetan	2nd generation for community acquired pneumonia; 2 g, IV BID
Cefoxitin	3rd generation, 2 g 6 hourly IV
Cefpirome	4th generation cephalosporin, 1–2 g IV BID
Cefpodoxime	3rd generation cephalosporin, 200 mg PO BID
Cefprozil	2nd generation for community acquired pneumonia, 500 mg PO BID
Ceftaroline	5th generation for MRSA and gram–negative organism, 600 mg IV BID/TID
Ceftibuten	3rd generation, 400 mg PO daily
Ceftazidime	Broad spectrum; 2 g IV TID
Ceftizoxime	Broad spectrum; 1–2 g IV BID/TID
Ceftriaxone	Third generation; 2 g IV TID
Cefuroxime	2nd generation, commonly for community acquired pneumonia, 500 mg PO BID

1st generation	*2nd generation*	*3rd generation*	*4th generation*	*5th generation*
Cefazolin	Cefamandole	Cefoperazone	Cefepime	Ceftaroline
Cefadroxil	Cefuroxime	Cefotaxime	Cefpirome	
Cefalexin	Cefaclor		Ceftazidime	
	Cefprozil		Ceftriaxone	
		Cefdinir		
	Cefoxitin	Cefixime		
	Cefotetan		Cefpodoxime	
			Ceftibuten	

Cefditoren	Broad spectrum cephalosporin; 200 mg PO BID
Celecoxib	Non narcotic analgesic, useful for gout, OA 100–200 mg PO BID
Celeprolol	Beta blocker, 200 mg 1–3 times daily
Cephalexin	Cephalosporin for skin infection, cellulitis; 250–500 mg PO QID
Ceritinib	Tyrosine kinase inhibitor for metastatic lung cancer (NSCC)
Cerivastatin	Statin for hyperlipidemia
Certolizumab	Anti TNF antibody for Crohn's disease, rheumatoid arthritis, 400 mg SC at 0, 2, 4 weeks; then 200 mg every other week
Cetirizine	Antihistamine, 5–10 mg OD
Cetrorelix	GNRH receptor antagonist 0.25 mg SC daily for precocious puberty
Cetuximab	EGRF antagonist used for colorectal cancer, squamous carcinoma, head and neck cancer; Dose 450 mg/m^2 IV loading; then 250 mg/m^2 IV weekly
Chlorambucil	Anti neoplastic alkylating agent, for CLL, NHL, HL; 5 mg PO daily

Chloramphenicol	Inhibits bacterial protein synthesis, used in enteric fever, meningococcal disease, plague, relapsing fever, scrub typhus, tularemia, Whipple disease; 250–500 mg 6 hourly
Chlordiazepoxide	Benzodiazepine used in anxiety, alcohol withdrawal
Chlorhexidine	Antiseptic for mouth wash, skin disinfection
Chlorphenothane	For typhus fever
Chloroadenosine	For cancer, HCL
Chloroquine	Used for malaria prophylaxis, *P. vivax*, SLE, porphyria cutanea tarda, Whipple disease;
Chlorproguanil	Antimalarial
Chlorpheniramine	Antiallergic, 25 mg TID
Chlorpromazine	Benzodiazepine for delirium, adjunct in schizophrenia, 100–1000 mg/day
Chlorthalidone	Diuretic for heart failure, IHD
Chlorpropramide	Oral anti diabetic agent; 100–500 mg OD
Chlorothiazide	Diuretic, up to 500 mg BID
Chymopapain	Injected for herniated disc
Cholestyramine	Used in hyper lipidemia, IBS and for pruritus of hepatic dysfunction
Ciclopirox	Agent for dermatophytosis
Cidofovir	Anti viral for CMV, HSV; 5 mg/kg IV once a week
Cilastatin	Renal dihydropeptidase inhibitor, combined with carbopenem
Cilansetron	5 HT receptor modulator for IBS, nausea and vomiting
Cilnidipine	Anti hypertensive; 5–20 mg OD
Cilazapril	For hypertension

Cilostazol	For claudication, antiplatelet, fibrinolytic 100 mg PO BID
Cimetidine	Inhibits gastric acid secretion; used in GERD, peptic ulcer, gastrinoma; 400 mg BID
Cinacalcet	Calcimimetic agent for reduction in PTH and hence serum calcium
Cinnarizine	Vasodilator for vertigo; 25 mg PO TID
Ciprofloxacin	Quinolone antibiotic for cholera infection, clostridia, enteric fever, plague, legionella, infectious diarrhea; 500 mg PO BID
Cisapride	Used in IBS, now withdrawn
Cisplatin	Platinum compound for gastric, cervical, bladder, hepatic, lung, bone testicular cancer; 50–100 mg/m^2 IV every 3–4 weeks
Cisatracurium	Neuromuscular blocker, used in ventilator therapy
Clozapine	Antipsychotic, 150–600 mg/day
Clomipramine	Anti depressant 150–300 mg/day
Chlorazepate	For epilepsy, anti anxiety; 15 mg
Citalopram	Anti depressant, often used in IBS, 20–60 mg/day
Cladribine	Antineoplastic agent, used in AML; 0.09 mg/kg/day IV infusion
Clarithromycin	Macrolide antibiotic, used in CAP, legionella, *H. pylori* 250–500 mg PO BID
Clavulanate	Beta lactamase inhibitor, combined with ampicillin and amoxicillin
Clemastine	Antiallergic, 1 mg BID PO
Clindamycin	Antibiotic for pelvic infections, skin infections; 300–450 mg PO
Clofazimine	Antileprotic agent, 50 mg daily
Clomipramine	Tranquilizer, sedative, 150–300 mg/day
Clofazimine	Used in leprosy, MDR/XDRTB;

Clonazepam	Anti anxiety sedative, 0.25 mg, 1–3 times daily
Clobazam	Anti epileptic, 16–40 mg/day
Clenobuterol	A sympathomimetic, bronchodilator
Clofarabine	Antimetabolite, for childhood ALL, 52 mg/ m^2 IV daily for 5 days
Clonidine	Used for smoking cessation, HTN; 100 μg tab TID; patch
Clorthalidone	Thiazide diuretic; 25–50 mg OD
Clorpromazine	Neuroleptic, dose 25–50 mg PO, IM, IV 4–12 hourly
Chlordia- zepoxide	Antianxiety agent; 10 mg PO
Codeine	Morphine derivative, analgesic, sedative, cough suppressant; reduces gut motility, 30–60 mg 4–6 hourly
Clopidogrel	ADP receptor antagonist for CAD, 75 mg PO OD
Cortisol	Steroid hormones of adrenal grand
Colistin	Polymixine for Pseudomonas; 5 mg/kg IV loading then 3 mg/kg/day in two divided doses, also oral suspension
Clomiphene	For ovulation induction; 25, 50 mg tab
Chlorthiazide	Diuretic 5–2 g daily in 2 divided doses
Ciclesonide	Inhaled corticosteroid prodrug for asthma
Clonazepam	Anti anxiety, 1–12 mg/day, also for schizophrenia
Clotrimazole	Systemic, local use antifungal, 100 mg/200 mg tab/lozenges
Clopamide	Diuretic for CHF, HTN, 5–30 mg/daily
Crizotinib	ALK, ROS inhibitor for NSCLC, anaplastic large cell lymphoma

Cloxacillin	Antibiotic, used with ampicillin; cap/inj; for RTI
Cromolyn sodium	Used in bronchial asthma as inhalation for short term benefit
Cyclophos-phamide	Cytotoxic, direct DNA interacting agent used in CLL, bladder cancer, lupus nephritis, MM, pemphigus vulgaris, TTP, systemic sclerosis, 500 mg IV every 2 weeks with mesna
Clozapine	Antipsychotic, 25/100 mg tab
Cycasin	A toxic substance of food causing ALS, dementia
Cyclandelate	Smooth muscle relaxant; 200–400 mg Cap/Tab
Cycloserin	Analog of D analine, second line anti-tubercular 250 mg PO BID/TID
Cyclosporine	Calcineurin inhibitor, immune suppressant for post-transplant patients, SLE, psoriasis, myasthenia gravis, IBD, epidermolysis bullosa 2–4 mg/kg IV infusion
Cyproheptadine	Antiserotonin used in angioedema, carcinoid syndrome, urticarial, appetite stimulant, 2–4 mg TID PO
Cyproterone	Antiandrogen for hirsutism, polycystic ovary syndrome
Cytarabine	Anti neoplastic agent for AML, CNS lymphoma, mantle cell lymphoma 100; mg/m^2 IV daily
Cyclopentolate	Mydriatic 1% eye drop; for eye examination

D

Dabigatran	Direct thrombin inhibitor used in pulmonary thromboembolism, stroke prophylaxis/ VTE prophylaxis, 75–150 mg PO OD
Dabrafenib	BRAF inhibitor used in melanoma, lung cancer
Dacarbazine	DNA alkylator used in soft tissue sarcoma, malignant pheochromocytoma, melanoma; 220–375 mg/m^2 IV on day 1, 15
Daclatasvir	NS 5A inhibitor used in HCV, 60 mg PO OD
Darbepoetin alfa	Stimulates erythropoiesis 250 μg SC every month
Daglutril	Dual inhibitor of endothelin and neprilysin like fasudil
Dacilizumab	CD 25 antibody, now withdrawn
Dactinomycin	For cancer uterus, Wilms' tumor, Ewing sarcoma, 0.04 mg/kg IV weekly
Dalbevancin	Lipoglycopeptide antibiotic used in complicated skin and soft tissue infection, 1500 mg PO once
Dalfampridine	Extended release 4 amino pyridine for multiple sclerosis
Dalfopristin	Prevents protein synthesis (streptogramin group), useful in macrolide resistant group of organisms
Dalteparin	Anticoagulant for pulmonary embolism, 200 IU/kg OD
Danaparoid	A mixture of glycosaminoglycans with anti Xa activity, used in heparin induced thrombocytopenia

Danazol	For ITP, fibroid; Ca breast, SLE; endometriosis; 200–800 mg/day
Dantrolene	Direct muscle inhibitor for spasticity, hyperthermia; 25–50 mg; 20 mg/vial
Dapagliflozin	SGLT2 inhibitor for DM2; 5–10 mg BID/OD
Dapsone	Anti leprosy drug, also useful for acne vulgaris, for PCP prophylaxis, toxoplasmosis prophylaxis in HIV, dermatitis herpetiformis, mucous membrane permphigoid, epidermolysis bullosa, relapsing polychondritis; Dose 100 mg/day PO for 5 years in tubercular leprosy and life long in lepromatous leprosy
Daptomycin	Lipopeptide antibiotic against gram–positive organism; 6–8 mg/kg IV OD
Daraprim	Pyrimethamine; antimalarial also for toxoplasmosis, leishmaniasis
Daratumumab	CD 38 antibody for multiple myeloma; 16 mg/kg/week IV for 8 weeks
Darbepoetin alfa	Recombinant erythropoietin for anaemia of CKD, hypoproliferative anemia, 25–200 g IV
Darifenacin	For over active bladder, 7.5/15 mg tab
Darunavir	Anti retroviral agent, 600 mg bid
Daunorubicin	For leukemia, 0.5–3 mg/kg IV
Dasabuvir	Antiviral for HCV (NS 5A inhibitor)
Dasatinib	Tyrosin kinase inhibitor for ACL, CML
Daunorubicin	Used for AML, Kaposi sarcoma; 30–60 mg/m^2 IV daily for 3 days or weekly
Debrisoquine	Anti hypertensive agent
Decitabine	Antineoplastic agent for AML, myelodysplasia, sickle cell anaemia 20 mg/m^2 IV (0.5–3 mg/kg)
Deferasirox	Iron chelator for hemochromatosis, 25–35 mg/kg PO

Deferoxamine	Iron chelator for hemochromatosis, 500 mg IM; 15 mg/kg/hr IV
Deflazocort	Corticosteroid, very potent, for asthma, RA, SLE; 6, 24, 30 mg tab, 3–18 mg daily
Degarelix	GnRH antagonist for castration in prostate cancer; 240 mg SC
Decavirdin	Non nucleoside RTI, anti HIV
Delamanid	Second line antitubercular agent like pretonamid; 200 mg PO OD
Delafloxacin	For *S. aureus, S. pneumoniae*; 450 mg BID
Demeclocycline	A tetracycline antibiotic known to cause nephrogenic diabetes insipidus
Denileukin - diftitox	Immunotherapy for CTCL; 9–18 mg/kg/day IV on days 1, 5; then every 3 weeks
Denosumab	Increases bone density, used in postmenopausal osteoporosis; anti RANKL antibody
Desipramine	Antidepressant; 150 mg/day
Desirudin	Recombinant hirudin–direct thrombin inhibitor for clot lysis
Desloratadine	Antihistamine, 5 mg daily
Desmopressin (DDAVP)	Used an adult hypopituitarism, central diabetes insipidus, coagulation disorders in CKD, haemophilia, sleep enuresis, orthostatic hypotension, von Willebrand disease, platelet function disorder 10 μg/dose nasal spray
Desonide	Low potency corticosteroid, local application 0.05%
Dexamethasone	Glucocorticoid given in cerebral edema, raised ICP, spinal cord compression, 4 mg IV; 0.5 mg tab, ointment, eye drop
Dexfenfluramine	Appetite suppressant
Dexlansoprazole	PPI (proton pump inhibitor), 30 mg OD

Dexmedetomidine	Sedative, does not cause delirium unlike midazolam; 6 μg IV,
Dexamethasone	Potent steroid for raised ICT, shock; for up to 100 mg IV/day
Dexrazoxane	Intracellular ion chelator for reducing anthracycline toxicity; dose 10.1 ratio of anthracycline
Dextromethorphan	Centrally acting cough suppressant, 10 mg/dose
Dextroamphetamine	CNS stimulant, high abuse potential, causes hypertrichosis
Diacerin	For musculoskeletal pain, 50 mg OD
Diazepam	Anxiolytic, sedative, used in status epilepticus, dystonia, porphyria, tetanus; 2–5 mg 1–3 times daily
Diazoxide	A benzothiazide, often used in insulinoma, hypertensive crisis, 150–300 mg IV
Dicarbazine	Used in cryptosporidiosis
Dichloraphenazone	Used in Hodgkin's disease
Diclofenac	NSAID for pain, gout, arthritis, migraine, 1–3 mg/kg/day; 75 mg/3 ml inj.
Dicloxacillin	Antibiotic for gram–positive infection; 250–500 mg PO QID
Dicyclomine	Anticholinergic for IBS, antispasmodic, tab, drops, syrup inj –10 mg /ml
Didanosine (ddi)	Antiretroviral agent, 250–400 mg daily in 2 divided doses
Diethyl carbamazine	Drug for lymphatic filariasis, loiasis, tropical pulmonary eosinophilia; 100 mg TID
Diethyldithiocarbamate	For nickel poisoning
Diethylpropion	Antiobesity agent, sympathomimetic–adrenergic agent

Diethyl stilbestrol	Estrogen for prostate cancer, postcoital contraception, 50 mg tab
Diflunisal	Drug for ATTR amyloidosis, 500–1000 mg daily, also in rheumatoid arthritis
Digoxin, Digitoxin	Cardiac glycoside for heart failure, dose, 0.125–0.25 mg PO OD
Dihydro-artemisinin	Antimalarial agent, active metabolite of arteether, artesunate
Dihydro-ergotamine	For migraine, exercise headache, 1 mg tab; 1 mg IV/IM/SC; max. 3 mg/day; 6 mg/week; 0.5 mg nasal sprays.
Difluoro methylornithine	For trypanosomiasis
Diloxanide furoate	A substituted acetanilide for luminal EH cysts; 250 mg TID
Diltiazem	Antiarrhythmic used in hypertension, CAD, arrhythmias, atrial tachycardia, dose 30–60 mg PO 8 hourly, 0.25 mg/kg IV/m × m 20 mg
Dimenhydrinate	Antihistaminic for motion sickness, vertigo, inner ear disease; 50 mg OD/BID
Dimercaprol	Chelator for heavy metal poisoning like arsenic, cadmium, mercury
Dimethyl-fumarate	Drug with anti-inflammatory effect used in psoriasis and multiple sclerosis
Dimethyl-sulfoxide	Agent for bladder instillation in interstitial cystitis/BPH
Dimethyl-tryptamine	Mind alerting agent
Dinutuximab	Anti GD_2 for pediatric neuroblastoma
Diphenhydra-mine	Antiemetic used for anaphylaxis, vertigo, pruritus; taxane and radio contrast premedication; constituent of cough syrups—15 mg/5 ml

Dipyridamol	Used in essential thrombocytopenia, CAD; TIA, 50–100 mg PO OD
Diphenoxylate	Mild opiate for diarrhea; 2.5 mg tab, 2 tab TID
Diphenyl-hydantoin	Used to control hypoglycaemia of insulinoma uncontrolled with diazoxide
Divalproex	For epilepsy
Dipivefrin	Used for glaucoma
Disopyramide	Antiarrhythmic agent; dose 100–300 mg PO 8 hourly
Disodium-chromoglycate	Used in bronchial asthma
Disulfiram	Agent for promoting alcohol abstinence, 250 mg–500 mg daily
Divalproex sodium	Anticonvulsant, valproic acid congener
Dobutamine	Sympathomimetic for cardiogenic shock/septic shock, stress testing, 2–20 μg/kg/min infusion
Docetaxel	Mitotic spindle inhibitor used in cancer of bladder, breast, stomach, lung, prostate, 60–100 mg/m^2 IV every 3 weeks
Docosanol	Topical application for herpes simplex; 10% cream 5 times daily
Docusate	Purgative, 100 mg BID
Dofetilide	Class III antiarrhythmic for atrial flutter/fibrillation, ventricular arrhythmias; Dose 0.125–0.5 mg PO BID
Dolasetron	5 HT_3 blocker for vomiting of anticancer medication
Dolutegravir	Antiretroviral agent; 50 mg daily PO
Domperidone	Antiemetic, 10–30 mg per dose
Donepezil	Drug for Parkinson's disease and dementia; 5–10 mg OD

Dopamine	Sympathomimetic for septic shock, hypothermia, Parkinson's disease, migraine
Dorzolamide	Antiglaucoma; 2% eye drop TID
Doripenem	Carbapenem antibiotic for Pseudomonas, anaerobic infection
Doxazosin	α_1 adrenergic antagonist for hypertension, Raynaud's phenomenon 1–16 mg OD
Doxacurium	Neuromuscular blocker 1 mg/ml vial
Doxepin	For depression, pruritus, urticaria, angioedema, insomnia, 200 mg/day
Doxophylline	Bronchodilator 400 mg BID
Doxorubicin	Antitumor antibiotic for Ca bladder, breast, liver, lung, sarcoma, multiple myeloma; 60 mg/m^2 IV every 3 weeks
Doxycycline	Tetracycline antibiotic effective for typhus, Q fever, plague, Lyme disease, donovanosis, anthrax, Brucella and Chlamydia, 100 mg BID
Doxylamine	Antihistaminic, 10 mg tab, 2 HS
Dosulephin	Antidepressant
Drospirenone	An analog of spironolactone having anti-androgen and anti-mineral corticoid activity, used as progestational agent
Dronaderone	Antiarrhythmic; 400 mg PO BID
Drospirenone	A progesterone, often causes hyperkalemia
Droperidol	Used in migraine
Drotaverine	Antispasmodic, 40–80 mg TID
Droxidopa	Used for treatment of orthostatic hypotension associated with Parkinsnism, MSA
Dulaglutide	GLP 1, receptor agonist for diabetes mellitus; 0.75 mg SC weekly
Duloxetine	Antidepressant, also used for neuropathic pain, fibromyalgia; 40 mg/day

Durvalumab	PDL, PD-1 pathway inhibitor (immune check point inhibitors) for NSLC, urothelial cancer
Dutasteride	Used for prostate cancer prevention (5α reductase inhibitor) like finasteride, 0.5 mg daily
Diethyl-carbamazine	For filariasis, loiasis, 100 mg TID
Dydrogesterone	Progesterone for endometriosis, luteal insufficiency, recurrent miscarriage, dysmenorrhea; 10–30 mg daily

E

Ebastine	Antiallergic, 10–20 mg OD
Ecallantide	Kallikrein inhibitor for urticaria and angioedema
Econazole	For candidiasis, 1% cream
Eculizumab	Binds to complement C_5, used in treatment of paroxysmal nocturnal haemoglobinurea, myasthenia gravis, MPGN, postrenal/cardiac transplant
Edaravone	Employed in treatment of amyotropic lateral sclerosis, ishaemic stroke; 1.5 mg inj.
Edrophonium	For snake bite, 0.25 mg/kg
Edoxaban	60 mg OD PO in anticoagulation of venous thromboembolism
Eicosapentanoic - acid	For hypertriglyceridemia, 180 mg, 3–5 cap daily
Embramine	Antiallergic, 25 mg tab, 1–2 tab daily
Elixacaftor	CFTR modulator for cystic fibrosis
Efavirienz	Anti-HIV agent, 600 mg PO
Eflornithine	For *Pneumocystis pneumoniae*, trypanosomasis; 200 mg/kg BID for 7 days
Elbasvir	NS5A inhibitor for HCL; 50 mg OD
Eletriptan	5HT receptor agonist for migraine; 40–80 kg/day
Elotuzumab	Therapeutic agent for multiple myeloma; 10 mg/kg IV on days 1, 8, 15, 22
Eltrombopag	Oral drug for TTP, but romiplostim is parenteral
Eluxadoline	Opioid antagonist–agonist for diarrhea of IBS
Elvitegravir	Antiviral for HIV, only given in combination with tenofovir, 1 tab daily

Emetine	Used in amoebiasis and fasciolopsiasis; 1 mg/kg/IM daily
Empagliflozin	SGLT2 inhibitor for diabetes mellitus
Emtansine	Microtubule directed drug for cancer
Emtricitabine	Antiretroviral, used in combination with tenofovir; 200 mg QID
Enalapril	ACE inhibitor for hypertension, CHF, 2.5–20 mg BID
Enalaprilat	Parenteral ACE inhibitor for aortic dissection, hypertensive emergency, 0.625–1.25 mg IV, max. 15 mg/hour
Endostatin	A peptide of endothelial cells that inhibits angiogenesis
Enfuvirtide	Anti HIV agent, 90 mg SC BID
Enoxaparin	LMW heparin used in PCI, AMI and VT prophylaxis; 20 mg, 40 mg SC or 1 mg/kg SC
Entacapone	COMT inhibitor for Parkinsonism, 200 mg with each levodopa
Entecavir	Anti HIV agent, 0.5 mg/day PO
Enzalutamide	Androgen receptor blocker for prostate cancer
Epalrestat	Cerebral enhancer, 50–150 mg TID
Ephedrine	Used in nasal drops, hypotension, myasthenia, 15 mg PO
Epinephrine	Beta agonist for anaphylaxis, severe asthma, hypoglycemia and shock
Epirubin	Like doxorubicin; 60–100 mg/m² IV weekly
Eptifibatide	Gp IIb–IIIA antagonist used in PCI; 180 μgm/kg bolus, 2 doses then 2 μg/kg infusion
Eplerenone	Diuretic, aldosterone antagonist for CHF, HT; 25 mg OD
Eptinezumab	CGRP–binding agent for relief of migraine

Eplerenone	Aldosterone antagonist for HTN, CHF, 25–50 mg OD
Epoprostinol	Prostanoid for pulmonary hypertension given IV
Epratuzumab	Monoclonal linked to bacterial toxin for ALL
Eptifibatide	Antithrombotic used, in CAD; 180 μg/kg bolus 2 doses then 2 μg/kg/min infusion
Esomeprazole	PPI, 20 mg OD
Erdosteine	Expectorant, 300 mg BID
Erenumab	Monoclonal for CGRP receptor for treatment of migraine
Ergotamine	For migraine, exercise headache/post coitus headache, maximum 6 tab/day; 10 tab per week (1 mg tab)
Eribulin	Microtubule remodeling agent for cancer treatment, breast cancer
Erlotinib	Tyrosine kinase inhibitor for hepatic, pancreatic and lung cancer; 150 mg PO daily
Ertapenem	A carbopenem for gram–positive/–negative organism and anerobes, 1 g infusion daily
Ertugliflozin	$SGLT_2$ inhibitor for diabetes
Erythromycin	Macrolide antibiotic used for gram–positive coccal infection, chlamydia, cancroid, bacillary angiomatosis, diphtheria, donovanosis; 500–1000 mg PO BID
Erythropoetin (epoietin)	Used for hypoplostic anaemia of CKD and often orthostatic hypotension; 100–300 IU/kg SC three times a week
Escitalopram	Antidepressant, 10–30 mg/day
Esmolol	Beta blocker for hypertensive emergency, arrhythmia, IHD; 500 μg/kg IV over 1 minute
Estrogen	Female sex hormone, cardioprotective and maintains bone health but linked to breast cancer
Estradiol	Estrogen for anovulation

Estramustine	Antimicrotubule, 14 mg/kg PO daily for metastatic prostate cancer
Eszopiclone	Benzodiazepine receptor agonist, hypnotic
Etanercept	TNFR Fc fusion protein for rheumatoid arthrits, 50 mg SC weekly
Ethacrynic acid	Loop diuretic; 50–100 mg BID/TID
Ethambutol	Anti-tubercular agent, 15 mg/kg/day PO
Ethamsylate	Hemostyptic, 500 mg QID
Ethionamide	Anti-tubercular agent, 15–20 mg/kg daily
Etizolam	Anxiolytic, up to 3 mg daily
Ethosuximide	Antiepileptic agent; 20–40 mg/kg/day
Ethacridine	Extra-amniotic infusion for pregnancy termination
Etidronate	Bisphosphonate for osteoporosis, hyperkalemia; 200–400 mg PO daily
Etodolac	NSAID, 600–1000 mg daily
Etomidate	Hypnotic–short acting, used for intubation
Etoposide	For lung cancer; NHL, HD, 100 mg/m^2 IV daily for 5 days or 50 mg/m^2 PO daily for 21 days in SCLC
Etravirine	NNRTI for HIV, 200 mg BID
Etoricoxib	NSAID, 90 mg BID PC
Etretinate	For psoriasis, Vit A analog
Everolimus	mTOR inhibitor, anticancer agent, immunosuppressant, used in cardiac transplant
Evolocumab	PCSK9 inhibitor for hyperlipidemia, 140 mg 2 weekly
Exemestane	Aromatase inhibitor for breast cancer, 25 mg daily
Exenatide	Long acting GLP 1, receptor agonist for DM, 200 μg pen, SC
Ezetimibe	Cholesterol lowering agent, 10 mg OD
Ezogabine	Potassium channel facilitator for epilepsy
Estramustine	For Ca prostate, 140 mg cap 4–6 cap daily

F

Famciclovir	Antiviral for HSV, HZV; 500 mg PO TID
Famotidine	PPI for gastritis, peptic ulcer, 40 mg OD
Faropenem	Imipenem group antibiotic; 200 mg PO TID
Felbamate	Anticonvulsant–sedative–hypnotic; 2400–3600 mg/day
Felodipine	Calcium channel blocker for hypertension, 5–10 mg OD
Febuxostat	Uricosuric antigout, 40–80 mg OD
Fenfluramine	Used in general anxiety disorder
Fenmetrazine/-fendimetrazine	Appetite suppressant for obestity–25 mg OD
Fenofibrate	Fibrate hypolipidemic drug, 14.5 mg OD
Fenfluramine	Appetite suppressant; 120 mg OD
Fenoprofen	NSAID; 200 mg PO 4–6 hourly
Fentazine	Antihistamine for vertigo, 4 mg TID
Fentanyl	Morphine derivative, analgesic–sedative; transdermal patch 5–20 µg/hour
Fexofenadine	Antiallergic, 180 mg daily
Fidaxomicin	Antibiotic for *Cl–difficile*, 200 mg PO BID
Filgrastim, G-CSF	Colony stimulating growth factor for neutropenia of chemotherapy, 5 µg/kg/day SC
Pegfilgrastim	6 mg SC
Finasteride	Anti-androgen for prostate cancer prevention, androgenic alopecia, hirsutism, 1 mg daily
Fingolimod	Sphingosine-1 phosphate inhibitor for multiple sclerosis
Flavoxate	Urinary sedative, soothing agent, 200 mg TID
Flacainide	Anti-arrhythmic agent; 50–200 mg PO BID

Flaviperavir	Antiviral for COVID–19, H1N1, 1800 mg BID on day 1 then 800 mg BID
Filbanserin	Serotonin receptor agonist, increases sexual desire in women
Floxuridine	Antimitotic for metastatic GI cancer; 0.1–0.6 mg/kg/day through hepatic artery
Fluconazole	Antifungal for *Candida*, coccidiodes, *Cryptococcus*; 12 mg/kg loading then 6 mg/kg/day
Flucytosine	Antifungal, converted to 5 fluorouracil inside fungus–used in *Candida* endocarditis, cryptococcal meningitis; 100 mg/kg/day
Fludarabine	Anticancer agent for CLL, NHL; 25 mg/m^2 IV daily for 5 days
Fludrocortisone	Steroid used in SIADH, adrenal insufficiency, orthostatic hypotension
Flumazenil	Benzodiazepine antagonist
Flunarizine	For hypnic headache, migraine prophylaxis, 5–10 mg daily
Fluocinolone	Medium potency locally used steroid, 0.2%
Fluocinonide	High potency locally used steroid
Flucloxacillin	For *Staph aureus*, 2 g IV QID
Fluroquinolones	Antibiotics inhibiting DNA gyrase and topoisomerase IV, also used in MDR TB
Flurodeoxycerine	Anticancer agent
5 fluorocuracil	Anti-cancer agent, for GI cancer, breast cancer hepatoma, ovarian cancer; 500 g/m^2 IV weekly
Fluoxetine	Antidepressant, 10–80 mg/day
Fluoxymes-terone	Oral testosterone, 17 α- alkylated derivative for hypogonadism, prostate cancer; 2–10 mg PO daily

Flupenthixol	For depression, 0.5/1 mg tab; for schizophrenia 3 mg tab
Flufenazine	High potency first generation antipsychotic, 1–20 mg/day
Flurazepam	Anixiolytic, 15 mg/day
Flutamide	Non steroid antiandrogen, 250 mg PO TID
Fluvastatin	Hypolipidemic agent, 20–80 mg daily
Fluticasone	Steroid for allergy, nasal spray, inhaler, accuhaler
Fluvoxamine	Used for obsessive compulsive disorder, antidepressant, 100–300 mg/day
Folinic acid	Used for pancreatic cancer, methotrexate toxicity prophylaxis
Folistatin	A binding protein that binds activin
Follitropin-alfa	For anovulation; 75–150 IU (FSH)
Fomepizole	Ethylene glycol antagonist (alcohol dehydrogenase inhibitor), 1 mg IV
Fomivirsen	Antisense oligonucleotide for CMV retinitis, intravitreal, 330 mg day 1 and 15
Fondaparinox	Anticoagulant for CAD, VT, pulmonary embolism; 25 mg SC daily
Foscarnet	Antiviral for CMV, HSV, HHV-6 and viral encephalitis; 60 mg/kg 8 hourly IV
Formoterol	Selective beta agonist, for bronchial asthma, 6 μg rotacap
Fosamprenavir	Anti-retroviral agent, 700–1400 mg PO TID
Fosfomycin	Antibiotic for UTI, *A. baumannii*, citrobacter infection, 3 g single dose sachet BID
Fosphenytoin	Antiepileptic, 75 mg/ml IM/IV
Fosfestrol	For prostate cancer 300 mg/5 ml, 600–1200 mg daily IV
Fosinopril	ACE inhibitor, for CHF, 10/20 mg tab TID

Framycetin	Antibiotic for local application, oint/eye drop
Frovatriptan	Anti-migraine, 2.5–5 mg/day
Fulvestrant	Anti-estrogen for breast cancer treatment; dose 250 mg IV monthly
Fumagilin	Used in microsporidiasis
Furazolidine	Intestinal local antibacterial agent, also used for *H. pylori*, 100 mg tab 4 times daily
Furosemide	Loop diuretic for heart failure, pulmonary edema, HT, SIADH; 20–240 mg daily
Fusidic acid	Local antibacterial agent
Fostemsavir	Anti HIV (experimental)

G

Gabapentin	Anticonvulsant, also used for cluster headache, fibromyalgia, migraine, neuropathic pain, 900–2400 mg/day
Gadolinium	MRI contrast, can cause nephropathy
Galantamine	Reversible acetylcholine esterage inhibitor used for Alzheimer disease, 12 mg tab
Galcanezumab	MC antibody for migraine
Galidesvir	Antiviral for Ebola, other filo viruses
Galium nitrate	Used in hypercalcemia, reduces plasma calcium by decreasing bone resorption; dose—200 mg/m^2 IV daily
Ganciclovir	Antiviral for CMV, 5 mg/kg IV BID
Garenoxacin	For CAP, 200 mg tab, 2 tab daily
Gatifloxacin	Antibacterial, also used in MDR TB; 0.3% eye drop
Gefitinib	Tyrosine kinase inhibitor for head and neck cancer, 250 mg PO OD
Gemcitabine	Cytosine derivative for cancer of lung, breast, pancreas; dose—100 mg/m^2 every week
Gemfibrozil	A fibrate, reduces triglyceride level, 600 mg BID
Gemifloxacin	Quinolone used in CAP and gonococcal infection; 320 mg OD
Gemigliptin	A gliptin for diabetes mellitus, dipeptidyl peptidase inhibitor
Gemtuzumab	Biologic for solid cancers, causes tumor lysis syndrome; 9 mg/m^2 2 doses 2 weeks apart
Gentamicin	Aminoglycoside antibiotic for gram–positive and –negative infections, brucella, listeria, plague, PID; 80 mg IM TID

Glatiramer acetate	Composed of alanine, glutamic acid, lysine and tyrosine, moderately effective in multiple sclerosis; 20 mg SC daily
	Sulphonylureas for treatment of diabetes mellitus (insulin secretagogues)
Gilclazide	80–240 mg/day
Glimepiride	1–8 mg/day
Glipizide	2.5–30 mg/day
Gliquidone	30–80 mg/day
Glyburide	1.25–5 mg/day
Glycopyrolate	Belladonna derivative, often used in place of atropine in intubation; 0.2 mg/ml/inj; 1, 2 mg tab
Glucagon	1 mg injection for hypoglycemia
Gonadotropin	HCG, 2000/5000 IU/inj. for infertility, male hypogonadism
Golimumab	Anti IgG, antibody used for ankylosing spondylitis, rheumatoid arthritis, IBD, psoriasis, 50 mg SC every 4–8 weeks
Goserilin	LHRH agonist for prostate cancer, dose 3.8 mg SC every month
Gramicidin	Locally applied anti-bacterial agent
Granisetron	5 HT_3 receptor antagonist for nausea like palanosetron, dolasetron, tropisetron, ramosetron, 1, 2 mg tab, also injection 1 mg/ml
Grazoprevir	NS5A inhibitor for HCV; 100 mg OD
Griseofulvin	For dermatophytosis, mucocutaneous candidiasis, systemic photosensitizer; 125 mg/250 mg tab OD
Guanabenz	For hypertension, centrally acting
Guanethidine	Vasodilator, used for hypertension; 10–50 mg PO daily
Guanfacine	Alfa agonist for tics, hypertension, 0.5–2 mg OD

H

Halofantrin	An antimalarial, like lumefantrin; 500 mg PO 3 doses
Halcinonide	High potency locally acting steroid, used as ointment
Halofantrine	Amino alcohol, used for malaria
Haloprogin	For skin fungal infections
Haloperidol	High potency 1st generation antipsychotic; 0.5–5 mg PO, IV, IM 4–8 hourly
Halothane	Inhaled anesthetic
Heparin	Anticoagulant, 75 units/kg bolus then 20 IV/kg/hour infusion; 5000 IU BID for DVT prophylaxis
Heparinoid	Mucopolysaccharide polysulfate cream for superficial thrombophlebitis
Hydralazine	Antihypertensive for hypertension, pre-eclampsia, 37.5–75 mg TID PO; 10–50 mg IV every 90 min
Hydrocodone	Cough suppressant
Hydrocortisone	Local acting corticosteroids in skin creams, nasal drop, enema
Hydromorphone	Opioid for pain relief, 2–4 mg PO 6 hourly; 1–2 mg IM; also rectal
Hydroxychloroquine	Used for rheumatoid arthritis, SLE, Q fever, sarcoidosis, Whipple's disease, COVID-19, dose—200–400 mg/day orally
Hydroxyprogesterone	250/500 mg inj; in threatened abortion, premature labor

Hydroxyurea	Cytotoxic agent used in CML, thrombocytosis, sickle cell disease; 500–1500 mg/day orally
Hydroxyzine	Antihistamine used for angioedema, urticaria, mastocytosis, 10/25 mg tab, syrup
Hydroquinone	For skin pigmentation, local application; 25 mg HS
Hylan	For injection into knee/hip in osteoarthritis weekly × 3
Hyoscine-butylbromide	10 mg cap for biliary/GI colic

I

Ibalizumab	For multidrug resistant HIV-1; 2000 mg loading; then 800 mg 2 weekly
Ibandronate	Bisphosphonate for osteoporosis, 150 mg tab, monthly
Ibritumomab	Anti CD2 (conjugate with Yttrium-20), for NHL, 0.4 mc/kg
Ibrutinib	Bruton's tyrosine kinase inhibitor for CLL, MCL
Ibuprofen	NSAID; 600–800 mg TID/QID
Ibutilide	Antiarrhythmic for AF, 1 mg IV over 10 min
Icatibant	Bradkinin receptor–antagonist for hereditary angioedema
Idrocilamide	For ALS
Idoxuridine	1% antiviral eye drop, 1 drop every hour for herpetic keratitis
Idarubicin	Anti-tumor antibiotic for CML, ALL, MDS, 1200 mg/m^2 IV on day 1–3; with cytarabine
Idarucizumb	Monoclonal antibody for dabigatran reversal
Idelalisib	Reversible P 13K inhibitor for CLL
Idoxyuridine	1% eye drop for herpetic keratitis
Ifosamide	Alkylating agent used for sarcoma and testicular cancer, 1 g vial IV daily × 5 days
Iloperidon	Second generation antipsychotic, 12–24 mg/day
Iloprost	Inhaled prostacycline for pulmonary artery hypertension
Imdevimab	Used along with casirivimab for COVID-19
Imatinib	TK inhibitor targeting Bcr Abl; used in CML, GIST, melanoma, AML; 400–600 mg PO daily

Imeglimin	Antidiabetic, 500–1000 mg orally daily
Imidopril	Antihypertensive, 5 mg, 10 mg tab/daily
Imipenem	Carbapenem antibiotic (broad spectrum) given with cilastatin; Dose 1 g IV TID
Imipramine	Antidepressant, also used for sleep enuresis, pain adjunct; 150–300 mg/day
Imiquimod	Antineoplastic agent for warts, melanoma, basal cell carcinoma, cutaneous leishmaniasis
Indacarterol	Akin to olodaterol, vilanterol, sympathomimetic for asthma (under trial)
Indapamide	Diuretic for hypertension, 1.5 mg SR tab/OD
Indinavir	Protease inhibitor for HIV, 400 mg, cap; 800 mg 8 hourly
Indomethacin	Anti-inflammatory, pain killer used in gout, nephrogenic diabetes insipidus, postprandial hypotension, postcoitus headache; 25–50 mg PO 8 hourly
Inebilizumab	Anti CD 19 for neuromyelitis optica
Infliximab	Anti TNF antibody for IBD, RA, psoriatic arthritis; 3 mg/kg IV infusion at 0, 2, 6 days then every 8 weeks
Ingenol mebutate	Local therapeutic agent to prevent malignant transformation of premalignant skin lesion
Inotuzumab	CD 22 antibody for ALL, B cell lymphoma
Interferon	For HBV, HCV, HDV, RCC, polycythemia, CML
Interferon alfa 2a	For chronic HIV, HDV, melanoma, 3–5 million units SC daily/3 times a week; intralesional for condyloma
Inferferon alfa 2b	For HBV, HCV, HDV, condyloma
Interferon beta 1a beta 1b	For multiple sclerosis
Interferon alfacon	9–15 μg thrice weekly for chronic HCV

Interferon gamma	For HIV, Q fever, T cell lymphoma, non-TB mycobacterial infection, HBV, HCV
Iodoquinol	For treatment of amoebiasis, balantidiasis and *D fragilis*
Ipilimumab	CTLA4 inhibitor, for metastatic melanoma
Irbesartan	Antihypertensive, 150/300 mg tab/OD
Irinotecan	A camptothecan for colon cancer, Ewing sarcoma, gastric and pancreatic cancer, 125 mg/m^2 IV weekly for 4 weeks (topoisomerase inhibitor)
Isavuconazole	Newer azole for invasive aspergillosis and mucormycosis; 200 mg 8 hourly × 6 doses then once daily
Isoprenaline	Adrenergic, 2 mg amp; for shock
Isradipine	Calcium channel blocker for coronary ischaemia–2.5–10 mg BID
Isotretinoin	For acne vulgaris, oral leukoplakia
Isovalcono-zonium	Broad spectrum antifungal
Isoniazid	Antitubercular agent, 5 mg/kg maximum 300 mg PO OD
Isotretinoin	Antiacne, 10, 20 mg cap
Isoprinosine	Useful in treatment of subacute sclerosing panencephalitis, 100 mg/kg/day
Isoproterenol	Used for asthma, primary pulmonary hypertension, 1 in 5000/inj.
Isosorbide-dinitrate	Coronary vasodilator; 10–40 mg PO; 80–120 mg SR tab, OD
Isosorbide-mononitrate	10, 20 mg tab, coronary vasodilator, BID
Isocarboxazid	Antidepressant, 20–60 mg/day
Isoxsuprine	Uterine relaxant, vasodilator, 10 mg tab, 2 tab TID

Itopride	GI motility enhancer, 50 mg tab TID
Itraconazole	Antifungal for candida, dermatophytes, molasses, talaromycosis; histoplasmosis, 250 mg PO OD/100–200 mg IV
Ivabradine	Slows heart rate, effective in heart failure, angina; 5–7.5 mg BID
Ivacoftor	CFTR modulation in cystic fibrosis
Ivermectin	Helpful in scabies, filariasis, ascariasis, oncocerciasis, strongyloidiasis, trichinosis, Covid-19; 6–12 mg tab/OD
Ixabepilone	Antimitotic agent, microtubule stabiliser for breast cancer
Ixazomib	Proteasome inhibitor for multiple myeloma; 4 mg PO on days 1, 8, 15
Ixekizumab	IL–17 antagonist for psoriasis; SC every 4 weeks

K

Kanamycin	Aminoglycoside antibiotic for MDR tuberculosis, 15–30 mg/kg/day IM, maximum 1 gm
Ketamine	Used for sedation during intubation, often abused, can be used for minor surgical procedure, 10 mg/50 mg amp; IM/IV
Ketanserin	5 HT_1 and 5 HT_2 receptor antagonist for carcinoid syndrome, HT and diarrhoea
Ketoconazole	Antifungal, can be used in seborrhoeic, dermatitis, Cushing syndrome, cutaneous leishmaniasis, male precocious puberty, tinea infection (shampoo) hypercalcemia; 200 mg tab; 1–2 tab daily
Ketorolac	Analgesic, 15–60 mg IM/IV; PO
Ketotifen	Antiallergic, 1 mg, tab, twice daily
Ketoprofen	NSAID; oral, rectal, patch; 20–50 mg TID

L

Labetalol	Beta blocker for hypertensive emergency, autonomic storm, 200–600 mg BID
Lacosamide	Antiepileptic 200–400 mg/day
Lactulose	Purgative (10 g) as enema in hepatic encephalopathy (200 g TID)
Lamivudine	Antiviral for HIV, HBV, 100 mg/day PO
Lamotrigine	Antiepiletpic, also used for trigeminal neuralgia, 150–500 mg/day
Lanatoprost	Antiglaucoma eye drop; 1 drop once daily
Laninamvir-octanoate	Neuraminidase inhibitor for influenza A
Lanreotide	Somatostatin analog for acromegaly, insulinoma, VIPoma
Lanatoprost	Eye drop for glaucoma, one drop once daily
Lansoprazole	Proton pump inhibitor for peptic ulcer disease, 30 mg OD
Lanthanum	Phosphate binder for hyperphosphetemia of CKD, 250–500 mg tab, 1.5–3 g day (NS5A inhibitor)
Lapatinib	Tyrosine kinase inhibitor for breast cancer; 250 mg tab, 1.25–1.5 g daily
Ledipasvir	Antiviral for HCV genotype Ia, Ib; 90 mg OD
Leflunomide	For RA, psoriatic arthropathy, SLE; 10–20 mg PO daily
Lenalidomide	For multiple myeloma, lymphoma, myelodysplasia; 5–25 mg PO daily
Lenvatinib	Tyrosine kinase inhibitor for RCC, hepatoma
Lercanidipine	Antihypertensive, 10 mg OD

Lesinurad	New uricosuric agent, like probenecid
Letermovir	Antiviral for CMV
Letrozole	Aromatase inhibitor for PCOD, breast cancer; 2.5 mg OD
Leucovorin	Chemo protective agent for colorectal cancer, pancreatic cancer, PCP prophylaxis, toxoplasma prophylaxis; 10 mg/m^2 PO/IM/IV; 1 mg OD PO in megaloblastic anaemia
Leuprolide (leuprorelin)	LHRH agonist like goseriline for prostate cancer; Dose 7.5 mg IM once a month
Levamisole	Anthelmintic for ascariasis, 50 mg/150 mg tab, 50 mg tab for child; 150 mg tab, for adult
Levamlodipine	Antihypertensive, 2.5–5 mg daily
Levetiracetam	Antiepileptic, often used for cyclic vomiting syndrome, myoclonus, 1–3 gm/day
Levorphanol	Synthetic opioid analgesic, morphine like action
Levobunolol	For glaucoma; eye drop, 1 drop twice daily
Levodopa	Dopa agonist used for parkinsonism, dystonia
Levofloxacin	Quinolone for *Chlamydia, Campylobacter, Legionella*, plague, tularemia, HACEK, pneumococcal infection, 500–750 mg daily
Levocetirizine	Antiallergic, 5 mg/OD
Levomilnacipran	Norepinephrine and serotonin reuptake blocker for depression, 40–120 mg/day
Levonorgestrel	Ovulation suppressant, contraceptive; 1 tab daily for 21 days
Levomenol	Oral spray for periodontitis, gingivitis
Levorphanol	Opioid agonist–antagonist
Levosimendan	Myocardial calcium sensitizer for CHF, 0.1 gm/kg/min infusion
Levosulpiride	For functional dyspepsia, 25 mg tab, 1 tab BID

Levothyroxin	Thyroid hormone for replacement in myxedema, hypothyroidism, 25–200 mg daily
Licorice	Contains glycyrrhizic acid, a natural sweetner
Lidocaine	Local anaesthetic for topical anaesthesia, can be used for arrhythmia 1–3 mg/kg IV
Lidoflagine	60 mg tab, 1 to 3 tab daily for CAD
Linaclotide	Guanylate cyclase agonist for IBS, IV for arrhythmias, bladder irrigation
Lincomycin	300 mg/ml inj; for URTI
Linagliptin	DPP4 inhibitor for diabetes, 5 mg tab 1 daily
Linezolid	Oxazolidinones like tedizolid for CAP, MRSA infection, 600 mg twice daily PO; also infusion
Linifanib	Used for therapy of HCC
Liraglutide	GLP analog for diabetes mellitus, obesity; 1.8 mg OD
Lisinopril	ACE inhibitor; 10–40 mg OD
Lithium	For bipolar disorder, cluster headache; 400–800 mg/day
Lixisenatide	Short acting GLP-1 receptor agonist for diabetes, 10 mcg SC daily
Lobeline	Plant alkaloid used in antismoking preparation
Lofexidine	Alfa adrenergic agonist for opium detoxification
Lomitapide	Inhibitor of MTP for reducing LDL–VLDL, 5 mg OD
Lomefloxacin	400 mg tab, 1 daily for UTI, URTI
Lomustin (CCNU)	For treatment of astrocytoma, 130 mg/m^2 PO every 6 weeks
Lonafarnib	Antiviral for hepatitis D, 100 mg PO daily
Loperamide	Antimotility agent for diarrhea, IBS; 2 mg tab, TID

Lopinavir	Antiviral protease inhibitor for HIV, 200 mg twice daily
Loracarbef	2nd generation cephalexin, 200–400 mg PO BID
Loratadine	Antiallergic 10 mg tab, OD
Lorazepam	Benzodiazepine for anxiety, insomnia, delirium; 0.5–2 mg 4 hourly IM, IV, PO
Lorcaserin	Selective $5HT_2$ agonist for obesity, anorexiant, 10–20 mg daily PO
Lornoxicam	NSAID, 4, 8 mg tab, 1 tab twice daily
Losartan	Angiotensin receptor blocker for hypertension, heart failure, 50–150 mg OD
Loxapine	Antipsychotic (mid potency), 30–100 mg/day
Lurasidone	Second generation antipsychotic, 40–80 mg/day
Lovastatin	Statin for hyperlipidemia, 20–80 mg daily
Lumefantrine	For malaria, 120 mg (along with artemether 20 mg) 4 tab start
Lumacaftor	CFTR modulation agent for cystic fibrosis
Lubiprostone	For IBS, constipation, 2 mg twice daily
Loteprednol	Eye drop for seasonal conjunctivitis 4 times daily
Luliconazole	Antifungal, 1% cream
Luvistin	Antiallergic, 20 mg tab BID

M

Macitentan	Endothelin receptor antagonist for pulmonary hypertension, 10 mg PO OD
Macrolide	Antibiotic like azithromycin, clarithromycin, erythromycin
Mafenide acetate	Used topically for electrical wound injury
Malathion	Organophosphorus influencing cholinesterase
Maprotilin	TCA antidepressant, 25–150 mg/day
Maraviroc	Antiviral agent for HIV, binds to CCR5; 150–600 mg BID
Mannitol	20% infusion for cerebral edema
Maribavir	Benzoimidazole for CMV, EBV
Mazindol	Sympathomimetic anorexic agent for obesity
Mebendazole	Benzimidazole, deworming agent effective in hook worm, round worm, trichuris, trichinella; 100 mg PO
Mebeverine	Antispasmodic, 135 mg tab BID
Meclizine	Antihistaminic, also used for vomiting of pregnancy, 25–50 mg TID PO
Meclofenamate	Halogenated anthralinic acid for RA
Mecasermin	Recombinant human IgF1 for dwarfism, SC
Medroxalol	Beta receptor antagonist like carvedilol
Medroxy-progesterone	Long acting progesterone for perimenopausal bleeding, contraception, PCOD
Mechlorme-thamine	Alkylating agent for HD, NHL; 6 mg/m^2 IV on days 1 and 8
Mefenamic acid	Analgesic, 250, 500 mg tab; for pain, pyrexia
Megaldrate	Antacid, antireflux agent, 2 tab TID

Mefloquine	Antimalarial, for prophylaxis and treatment, 250 mg weekly for prophylaxis; 15 mg/kg followed by 10 mg/kg after 6 hours for treatment
Megestrol	Used for HIV and cancer related cachexia, 40, 160 mg tab; for cancer cachexia 40–320 mg daily
Meglumine-antimoniate	For leishmaniasis, 20 mg/kg IV daily for 30 days
Melatonin	Pineal hormone used to treat jet lag and to induce sleep, 9–12 mg daily tab/spray
Melarsoprol	For trypanosomiasis, 2.2 mg/kg IV for 10 days
Melphalan	Alkylating agent for multiple myeloma; 2–5 mg tab, 0.25 mg/kg/day for 4 days
Menaquinons	Vit K_2, synthesized by bacterial flora
Memantine	For dementia, 5, 10 mg tab, 5 mg daily
Mephenytoin	Antiepileptic, akin to ethotoin, 100 mg tab
Mepolizumab	IL-5 antagonist for eosinophilia
Mepacrine	Antimalarial, 100 mg, 300 mg tab; for prophylaxis
Meprobamate	Tranquiliser, muscle relaxant
Mercaptoethanesulfonate	(MESNA) Bladder protective from cyclophosphamide
6 Mercaptopurine	Drug for ALL; 50 mg tab; 2–5 mg/kg wt daily
Meropenem	For Pseudomonas, Klebsiella, Acenetobacter, 1 g IV TID
Mesna	Sulfhydryl compound for prevention of cyclophosphamide and ifosamide induced haemorrhagic cystitis; dose equivalant to ifosamide/cyclophosphamide
Mesalazine	4 g enema, 400 mg tab for ulcerative colitis; up to 2 tab TID

Meropenem–veborbactam	Carbopenem antibiotic effective against anaerobes CAP, Pseudomonas, *A. baumani*, MDRTB, whipple disease
Mesulphen	Locally acting antiscabies agent
Metanephrine	Sympathomimetic, increased in pheochromocytoma
Mesalamine	5ASA for IBD; 2.4–4.8 gm/day
Metaxalone	Muscle relaxant, 400 mg tab
Metformin	Antidiabetic for NAFLD, DM, PCOD; 500–2000 mg daily
Methadone	Morphine derivative for pain management and opioid withdrawal, 5–10 mg IM; 5–20 mg PO 6–8 hourly
Methamphetamine	Psychostimulant
Mesterolone	For androgen deficiency, 25 mg TID
Methaqualone	Addictive analgesic, 250 mg tab, with diphenhydramine
Metamizol	Analgesic, 500 mg tab
Methicillin	Old staphylococcal antibiotic
Methdilazine	For allergy, pruritus, 4 mg tab twice daily; syrup
Methimazole	Antithyroid drug, 5–10 mg tab, 50–60 mg daily
Metoclopramide	Antiemetic, 10 mg tab, syrup, inj; for gastritis, gastric hypotonia, duodenitis
Methocarbamol	Muscle relaxant, 350 mg tab TID
Methotrexate	Dihydrofolate reductase inhibitor for ALL, breast cancer, psoriasis, RA, SLE, vasculitis, IBD, MS, 10–25 mg weekly with folic acid
Methoxsalen	10 mg tab for vitiligo, psoriasis; 0.6 mg/kg alt days, then exposure to UV light
Methyl dopa	Vasodilator for HTN, 250–500 mg BID, PO, 500 mg IV

Methyl - ergometrine	For postpartum bleed; 200 mg TID
Methyl naltrexone	Peripherally acting opioid antagonist
Methyl-phenidate	Psychostimulant for depression, ADHD, fatigue, narcolepsy, 10 mg tab; 10–60 mg daily
Methylpred-nisolone	Corticosteroid for transplant rejection, anaphylaxis, gout, arteritis, IBD, MS, SLE, serum sickness, 40 mg/ml inj; 40–80 mg weekly
Methysergide	No longer manufactured, was used for migraine
Metoclopramide	Antiemetic, 10 mg tab; 5 mg/ml inj
Metolazone	Diuretic, 2.5/5 mg tab; OD
Metoprolol	Beta blocker for CAD, hypertension, arrhythmia; 5 mg IV for arrhythmia, 25–100 mg PO 6 hourly
Metrifonate	Drug for schistosmiasis, 3 doses at 2 weeks interval
Metronidazole	Imidazole for amoebiasis, anaerobes, bacterial vaginosis, Vincent angina, giardia, clostridia, PID, 400 mg PO TID, also IV inj
Metyrapone	Compound for pituitary function testing
Mexilentine	Antiarrhythmic, also used for pain, neuropathy; 150–300 mg PO TID
Methenamine	Urinary antiseptic
Mezlocillin	Extended spectrum penicillin
Mibefradil	Antipseudomonal penicillin
Milcafungin	Echinocandin for fungal infection, mainly candida, 400 mg PO/IV
Miconazole	Azole antifungal for candida, local acting, topical, vaginal
Midazolam	Sedative–anxiolytic for delirium, status epilepticus 1–5 mg infusion, SC/IM, PO, nasal

Midodrine	Alfa1 agonist for orthostatic hypotension, hepatorenal syndrome
Midostaurin	Multikinase inhibitor for mastocytosis, AML
Mifepristone	For postcoital contraception, 200 mg tab; also for pregnancy termination
Miglitol	Insulin secretagogue for DM; 25–100 mg daily
Minacipran	Balanced serotonin–norepinephrine receptor inhibitor for fibromyalgia; 25, 50 mg cap, max. dose 50 mg BID
Milrinone	Cardiac stimulant inotrope; up to 75 μg/kg/min infusion
Miltefosine	Drug for Naegleria, visceral leishmaniasis, trypanosomes; 2.5 mg/kg/day
Minocycline	Antibiotic for acne, actinomycosis, leprosy, legionella, skin infection, whipple disease, 100 mg PO BID
Minoxidil	Vasodilator for hypertension and local application for hair loss, 2.5 mg–5 mg OD/BID; 2%, 5%, 10% lotion
Mipomersen	Apo B inhibitor for VLDL reduction; 200 mg SC weekly
Mirtazapine	Anti-depressant, insomnia, and PML; 15–45 mg/day
Misoprostol	Used for acid peptic disease, as abortificient; 200 mg QID
Misonidazole	Neurotoxic amoebicide
Mizolastine	Anti-allergic; 10 mg tab. 1 daily
Mitiglinide	Non sulphonyl urea insulin secretagogue for DM
Mitomycin-C	Antitumor antibiotic, for breast, cervical, GI cancer and NSCLC; 10–20 mg/m^2 IV every 6 weeks
Mitotane	Adrenal steroidogenesis inhibitor for Cushing syndrome; 6–12 mg/day orally

Mitoxantrone	Synthetic compound for prostate cancer, multiple sclerosis, malignant pleural effusion Dose – 8–12 mg/m^2 IV every 3 weeks
Moclabemide	Antidepressant, 150, 300 mg tab; 300 mg daily
Modafanil	For depression, narcolepsy; 200–400 mg morning
Molgramostim	Recombinant GM CSF 150/300/450 mg for chemotherapy induced neutropenia
Molindone	Antipsychotic, 30–100 mg daily
Mometasone	Synthetic topical corticosteroid
Morizicine	Antiarrhythmic for atrial tachycardia
Morphine	Opioid analgesic for pain, AMI, pulmonary edema, sickle cell crisis; 5 mg IM/IV; 30 mg PO 4 hourly
Moxetumomab	CD22 antibody for ALL
Moxifloxacin	Quinolone, broad spectrum, 400 mg daily
Moxonidine	Centrally acting sympatholytic used for congestive heart failure, 300/200 mg tab/OD
Mupirocin	Locally acting antibiotic for staph infection, impetigo
Mycopheno-latemofetil	Purine synthesis inhibitor used in pemphigus, SLE, myasthenia gravis, lupus nephritis, post-transplant immune suppression 2–3 gm/day PO, maintanace 1–2 gm/day

N

N-acetyl cysteine	Used for paracetamol overdose, *H. pylori* eradication, prevention of contrast induced nephropathy
Nadroparin	Anti Xa; for AMI, DVT–2850 IU daily SC
Nabumetone	NSAID for osteoarthritis, rheumatoid arthritis
Nadifloxacin	Topical quinolone, 1% cream/lotion
Nadolol	Antiarrhythmic, also used in IHD, long QT syndrome; 40–240 mg/day
Nafamostat	Protease inhibitor for anticoagulation, pancreatitis
Nafarelin	To treat ovarian hyperandrogenism in PCOD; GnRH agonist like buserelin, goserelin, histrelin, leuprolide
Nafcillin	A penicillin useful for methicillin sensitive *Staph. aureus* like oxacillin, dicloxacillin and flucloxacillin, 1–2 g IV OD
Nafazolin	Conjunctival decongestant, 0.1 % eye drop
Nalidixic acid	Urinary antiseptic, 1 gm 6 hourly
Nalbuphine	Most potent analgesic better than pentazocine, 10 mg IM/SC
Nalfurafine	Opioid analgesic
Nalmefene	Opioid antagonist for alcohol deaddiction
Naloxone	Opioid antagonist 0. 4–2 mg IV/IM/SC for opioid, pentazocine, dextropropoxyphene over dose
Naltrexone	Opioid antagonist, 50 mg tab; 25–50 mg daily; used in alcohol rehabilitation 50–150 mg/day
Nandrolone	Anabolic steroid, 25 mg/ml inj.

Naproxen	Analgesic for pain, migraine, arthritis, dysmenorrhea, rheumatic fever; 375–500 mg BID
Naratriptan	5HT receptor agonist for migraine, 1 mg tab
Natalizumab	IgG_4 monoclonal for multiple sclerosis, Crohn's disease
Natamycin	Anti infective, 5% eye drop 4–6 times daily
Nateglinide	Non sulphonyl urea insulin secretagogue for DM; 60, 120 mg tab 1 tab before BF, lunch and dinner
Nebivolol	Cardio selective betablocker for CAD, HTN; 5–40 mg daily
Necitumumab	Monoclonal antibody against NSCL cancer targeting EGFR
Nedocromil-sodium	Chromone for bronchial asthma (mast cell stabilizer)
Nelfinavir	For HIV; 250 mg tab; 750 mg TID
Neomycin	Locally acting antibiotic
Nefazodone	5 HT_2 receptor modulator, antidepressant, 200–600 mg daily PO
Neostigmine	Acetylcholinesterage inhibitor for neurotoxic snake bite, myasthenia gravis; 0.01 mg/kg SC, IM, IV
Nepafenac	1 mg/ml eye drop, for pain relief, 1 drop TID
Neratinib	Ural tyrosine kinase inhibitor for breast cancer
Nesiritide	Vasodilator for acute heart failure; 2 μg/kg, IV bolus; then 0.01 μg/kg/min
Netazepide	Gastrin receptor antagonist for carcinoid
Netilmicin	Aminoglycoside antibiotic, 4–6 mg/kg IV/IM OD
Neumega (IL–II)	For chemotherapy induced thrombocytopenia, 50 μg/kg/day SC

Nevirapine	Anti HIV, 200 mg/day
Nicardipine	IV antihypertensive, 5 mg/hour, maximum 15 mg/hour
Nicorandil	Anti-angina; 10 mg twice daily
Nicumarol	For thromboembolism; 3–12 mg PO day 1, then 1–8 mg OD
Nifedipine	Calcium channel blocker for hypertension, CAD, 30–90 mg PO OD
Nifurtimox	Nitrofuran compound for typanosomiasis, 15 mg/kg/day, 3 doses
Nilotinib	Tyrosine kinase inhibitor for ALL, CML, 300 mg PO twice daily
Nilutamide	Antiandrogen, long acting; for metastatic prostate cancer; 300 mg PO daily
Nimesulide	NSAID, 100 mg tab, 1 BID, 3% gel/cream
Nimodipine	Calcium channel blocker, cerebral vasodilator, 20–40 mg OD; infusion
Nintedanib	Anti fibrotic agent for pulmonary fibrosis, 100 mg daily
Nelfinavir	Antiviral for HIV, 750 mg PO TID, or 1250 mg PO BID
Nitazoxanide	5 nitrothiazole, antiprotozoal for *Giardia, H. pylori, Cl. difficile, H. nana*; 500 mg BID × 3 day
Nitrazepam	For insomnia; 5–10 mg HS
Nitric oxide	Vasodilator–bronchodilator used in asthma, pulmonary hypertension
Nitrofurantoin	Bactericidal, for urinary tract infection, 100 mg PO BID
Nitroglycerin	Vasodilator, for angina, heart failure, cocaine toxicity; 20 μg/min, raised up to 200 μg/min; sublingual—3–6 mg; oral spray, transdermal patch, ointment; for hypertensive emergency—5 μg/min—20 μg/min infusion

Nitrendipine	Vasodilator, for hypertension, 10–20 mg OD
Nitrofurazone	Antibacterial, local use
Nitroimidazole	Delamanid is of this group for MDR-TB
Nitroprusside	Vasodilator for malignant hypertension, aortic dissection; 0.3 μgm/kg/min infusion
Nitrous oxide	Vasodilator for sickle crisis
Nivolumab	PD_1 antibody for HCC, RCC, HD, melanoma
Nizatidine	H_2 receptor antagonist for acid peptic disease, 300 mg OD
Nonoxynol	Spermicide in vaginal pessary
Norepinephrine	(Noradrenaline) beta agonist for hypotension, 4 mg/2 ml amp.
Norfloxacin	Quinolone for infectious diarrhea, donovanosis; 400 mg BID
Nomegestrol	Newer progesterone derivative
Normeperidine	Metabolite of meperidine causing seizure
Norgestrol	For DUB, endometriosis; 0.25 mg tab, 2–4 tab daily
Nortriptyline	Anti-depressant, also used for neuropathy, migraine prophylaxis, 50–200 mg/day
Nystatin	Anti-fungal, topical application
Noscapine	Anti-tussive, in cough syrup
Norethindrone	Progesterone for perimenopausal symptoms, 5 mg daily
Norethisterone	For menorrhagia; 5 mg tab, 1 tab BID/TID
Nylidrin	Peripheral vasodilator for thromboangiitis, claudication, 3–12 mg TID; 6 mg/ml inj. (for uterine relaxation)

O

Obinutuzumab	Anti CD2 antibody for CLL
Octinoxate	Constituent of sunscreen for UV induced hyperpigmentation
Ocrelizumab	Monoclonal antibody for multiple sclerosis
Octreotide	Somatostatin analog for acromegaly, gastrinoma, glucagonoma, insulinoma, somatostatinoma, Vipoma, ZES, carcinoid syndrome, 100–600 μg/day SC in two divided doses
Odalasvir	NS5A inhibitor for HCV
Odanacatib	Cathepsin k inhibitor for osteoporosis, under evaluation
Oestriol	1, 2 mg tab, maximum 4 mg in a week for estrogen lack of menopause
Ofatumumab	Anti CD20 for CLL
Ofloxacin	Quinolone for enteric fever, leprosy, plague, chlamydia; 200 mg BID; also eye/ear drop
Olanzapine	Antipsychotic, also useful in bipolar disorder; 2.5–5 mg QID/BID
Olaparib	ADP ribose polymerase inhibitor—for ovarian cancer
Olaratumab	PDGF-antibody for soft tissue sarcoma
OKT3	Human T cell antibody used for solid organ transplant
Olopatadine	Antiallergic; 5 mg twice daily; in nasal drop, ophthalmic ointment
Olmesartan	ARB for hypertension; 10, 20, 40 mg tab; 10–40 mg daily
Omacetaxine	Protein synthesis inhibitor for CML, 1.25 mg/m^2 SC BID × 14 days

Omalizumab	Anti IgE for asthma, urticaria; SC every 2–4 weeks
Omapatrilat	Endopeptidase inhibitor plus ACE inhibitor for heart failure
Omaveloxolone	Agent for treatment of mitochondrial DNA disease
Ombitasvir	Antiviral for HCV genotype Ia, Ib, IV, NSSA inhibitor
Omecamtiv	Inotrope for heart failure
Omeprazole	PPI for peptic ulcer disease, 20 mg OD
Ondansetron	$5HT_3$ receptor antagonist for nausea, vomiting, ataxia/tremor of MS, carcinoid syndrome, scombroid poisoning, 4/8 mg tab; 2 mg/ml 2 ml amp. for nausea, vomiting
Opicapone	COMT inhibitor for parkinsonism, 50 mg HS
Orciprenaline	Bronchodilator, syrup/10 mg tab for asthma
Orexin	The brain neurotransmitter for arousal
Oritavancin	Vancomycin related glycopeptide for MRSA, *S. pneumonia*, enterococci
Ornidazole	For giardiasis, amoebiasis; 500 mg BID
Orlistat	Derivative of lipase inhibitor lipostatin for obesity 60/120 mg Cap; 1 OD
Orphenadrine	Centrally acting muscle relaxant, for parkinsonism 50 mg TID
Oseltamivir	Antiviral for influenza, swine flu (treatment and prophylaxis), 75 mg PO BID
Osimertinib	Tyrosine kinase inhibitor for lung cancer with mutation (T 790 m)
Ospemifine	Hormonal agent to treat osteoporosis, postmenopausal genitourinary syndrome
Oxacillin	Penicillin for MSSA, endocarditis, cellulitis, osteomyelitis, dose –1–2 g IV QID
Oxaliplatin	Platinum analog for colon cancer, gastric cancer; 50/100 mg vial; 85 mg/m^2 every 2 weeks

Oxamniquine	Tetrahydroquinoline derivative for schistosomiasis, single dose orally
Oxazepam	Benzodiazepine for sedation, anxiety, 15 mg tab OD
Oxaprozin	For osteoarthritis, rheumatoid arthritis; 600 mg tab, 2 tab OD
Oxandrolone	Testosterone derivative given orally
Oxcarbamazepine	Anticonvulsant, for neuralgia and bipolar disorder, 300 mg PO TID; 900–2400 mg/day
Oxicam	NSAID group
Oxymetazoline	Locally acting vasoconstrictor, nasal drops for vasomotor rhinitis
Oxyphenoniumbromide	For gastritis, peptic ulcer, 5 mg tab; 1 tab 4 times daily
Oxycodone	Opium derivative for pain; 5–10 mg PO 4–6 hours
Oxyconazole	1% ointment for tinea
Oxyphenbutazone	NSAID
Oxprenolol	Antiarrhythmic 40/100 mg tab; 40–240 mg daily
Oxytocin	Posterior pituitary hormone, stimulates postpartum milk secretion
Oxybutynine	For urinary frequency/urgency, 2.5 mg TID
Oxytetracycline	250 mg cap; 4 cap daily, for respiratory infections, brucella, rickettsia

P

Paclitaxel	A taxane, mitotic spindle inhibitor for carcinoma breast, bladder, ovary, lung, melanoma, also in drug eluting stents. Dose – 80 mg/m^2 IV every week
Palbociclib	CDKS$_{4 \text{ and } 6}$ inhibitor for ER positive breast cancer
Palifermin	Keratinocyte growth factor for mucositis of radiation and chemotherapy, dose 60 μg/kg/day IV bolus
Paliperidone	Antipsychotic agent; 3–12 mg/day
Palivizumab	Monoclonal antibody for RSV prevention
Palonosetron	5HT$_3$ antagonist for nausea, vomiting of chemotherapy, 0.25 mg IV
Pamidronate	Reduction of hypercalcemia of bone metastasis, 90 mg IV every month, else 30 mg IV daily 3 days
Pancuronium	Neuromuscular blocking agent, 2 mg/ml inj. 50–100 μg/kg
Panobinostat	Histone deacetylase inhibitor for relapsed myeloma
Panitumumab	EGFR antagonist for colon cancer
Papaverin	Sympathomimetic, bronchodilator; inhaled in asthma
Pantoprazole	PPI for acid peptic disease, 40 mg PO/IV
Parcopa	10–25 mg tab for parkinsonism
Paracetamol	Analgesic, antipyretic, 500–2000 mg daily
Paritaprevir	For HCV genotype 1 and 4; 150 mg OD
Paroxetin	Antidepressant; 20–60 mg/day
Paromomycin	For amoebiasis, giardiasis, cutaneous leishmaniasis; 25–30 mg/kg/day PO

Pasireotide	Somatostatin analog, better than lanreotide and octriotide; for ACTH secreting pituitary tumor; 600–900 μg SC
Parecoxib	Pain killer; 40 mg injection twice to four times daily
Pasugrel	Antiplatelet for CAD; loading 60 mg PO then 10 mg daily
Pazopanib	VEGF inhibitor for RCC, soft tissue sarcoma
Pefloxacin	450 mg–tab, 400 mg infusion for gram–negative sepsis
Pegademase	Bovine adenosine deaminase; 250 IV/ml inj. for immunodeficiency states, SC ID
Pegfilgrastim	Depot preparation of G–CSF for neutropenia; 6 mg SC
Peg IFN alfa 2a	For HCV, HBV, HDV; 135 μg, 187 μg per 0.5 ml once weekly
alfa 2b	For HCV, HBV, HDV and melanoma
Pegloticase	IV use for hyperuricemia; 8 mg IV every 2 weeks
Pegvisomant	GH receptor antagonist for acromegaly; 10–20 mg IM daily
Parnaparin	A LMW heparin, 0.6 ml SC
Pazufloxacin	Atypical quinolone; 500 mg infusion twice daily
Pembrolizumab	PD1 antibody for NSC lung cancer, melanoma, HD, bladder cancer, Hodgkin's disease
Pemetrexed	Folate antimetabolite for lung cancer, 100/500 mg infusion
Pemoline	Non amphetamine psychostimulant, 18.75 mg BID
Penciclovir	Antiviral for HSV1, HSV3, VZV and EBV; also topical 1%
Penicillamine	Chelating agent for cystinuria, Wilson's disease, systemic sclerosis; 250 mg cap, maintenance dose 500–750 mg daily

Penicillin G Procaine, penicillin, penidure	For gram–positive organism, leptospirosis, anthrax, syphilis, Lyme disease, 6,00,000 units/vial; IM OD, 12, 00, 000 unit/vial (penidure)
Pentamidine	For PCP, cutaneous leishmaniasis, trypanosomiasis; 2–4 mg/kg IM daily for 2–7 days
Pentazocine	Narcotic analgesic, 15–30 mg TID PO; 30 mg/ml inj; 2 ml IM/IV
Pentid	Penicillin G; 2 lac, 4 lac, 8 lac unit tab; twice/thrice daily
Pentobarbital	Short acting barbiturate, sedative, hypnotic, given PO, rectal, parenteral
Pentosan-polysulfate	Semisynthetic polysaccharide for interstitial cystitis, bladder pain syndrome, 100 mg PO TID
Pentostatin	Cytotoxic antimetabolite for CLL, ALL given IV 4 mg/m^2 every other week
Pentoxy phylline	Used in alcoholic liver disease, claudication; 400 mg tab BID
Peramivir	Neurominidase inhibitor for influenza, 600 mg IV
Permethrin	Scabicide, applied locally
Pergolide	Used in hyperprolactinemia, ergot derivative; like cabergoline, quinagolide
Perindopril	4 mg tab, for hypertension
Pertuzumab	Anti HER_2 neu antibody for breast cancer
Phenacetin	Analgesic linked to cancer of bladder, rectum
Phenazo-pyridine	Urinary antiseptic, known to cause meth hemoglobinemia, 200 mg tab TID
Phencyclidine	Hallucinogen, intoxicant
Pheniramine	Antiallergic, anti-cold, up to 45 mg TID
Phenelzine	Antidepressant, used also in migraine prevention, 45–90 mg/day

Phenformin	Antidiabetic, causes metabolic acidosis, hence withdrawn
Phenytoin	Antiepileptic, 300–400 mg/day
Phenobarbital	Antiepileptic, sedative, 60–180 mg/day
Phenindione	For thromboembolic disorders; 50–150 mg PO OD
Phenoxy-benzamine	Used for detrusor/sphincter dys synergia, in HT, 20–120 mg BID–TID
Phentermine	Anorexiant for weight loss in obesity treatment; 10 mg morning 15 mg before meals
Phenylephrine	10% dye drop, mydriatic, cycloplegic, for uveitis, 1–2 drops; also in cough expectorants
Phentolamine	Vasodilator for adrenergic crisis due to cocaine, amphetamine; 5–15 mg bolus
Phenylbutazone	NSAID, can cause retinal bleed
Phenylephrine	Beta agonist, also 5% cycloplegic eye drop for uveitis, also in cough syrups
Phenytoin	Anticonvulsant; 100 mg tab, daily dose 200–600 mg; also used in trigeminal neuralgia
Pholcodeine	Cough suppressant, 1.5 mg/5 ml cough syrup
Physostigmine	Cholinergic agent for myasthenia, belladonna alkaloid over dose, mushroom poisoning, 2 tab TID
Pilocarpine	Cholinergic agent, for angle closure glaucoma, xerostomia, dry eyes, 1%, 2%, 4%, for glaucoma, 1–2 drops
Phytomenadione	10 mg/ml inj; antidote to coumarin anti-coagulant
Pimavanserin	Atypical neuroleptic, often used in PD
Pimecrolimus	Used as cream for atopic dermatitis, 10 mg/g cream

Pidotimod	400/800 mg tab, for prevention of COPD exacerbation
Pindolol	Cardioselective beta blocker; 2.5–7.5 mg TID
Pimozide	Diphenyl butyl piperidine class of anti-psychotic, 2, 4, 10 mg tab, max. 16 mg daily
Pioglitazone	Anti-diabetic agent, 15–45 mg daily
Piperacillin-(+tazobactum)	Antibiotic for CAP, GM–ve sepsis, anaerobic infection; 3.75–4.5 g IV 8–12 hourly
Piperaquine	Bisquinolone–antimalarial
Piperazine	Anthelminitic for ascariasis, 75 mg/kg PO (mxm 3.5 g)
Piracetam	Cerebral activator, 400/600 mg tab; also injection
Piribedil	For Parkinson's disease, 50 mg tab, 1–4 tab daily
Pirfenidone	Antifibrotic, used in pulmonary fibrosis like nintedanib; 200 mg TID to 600 mg TID
Pitavastatin	Hypolipidemic agent, 1–2 mg daily
Piroxicam	Analgesic, also used in colorectal cancer prevention; 20 mg tab; 40 mg injection; 0.5 % gel
Pivmecillinam	For UTI, 400 mg PO BID, Shigella– 100 mg QID
Pleconaril	Antiviral for picorna virus and rhinoviruses and enteroviruses
Pizotifen	Migraine prevention, 0.5–2 mg OD
Plerixafor	CXCR4 antagonist, used in bone marrow transplant
Plicamycin-(milthromycin)	Prevents bone resorption; in hypercalcemia 25 mcg/kg/day IV for 3 days
Pocapavir	Antiviral for enterovirus infection
Polymyxin B	For *P. aeroginosa* and *A. baumannie* but not gram–positive bacteria; 2.5–3 mg/kg/day IV in 2 divided doses

Polimyxin E	Colistin, as above but less neuro- and nephrotoxic
Pomalidomide	Related to thalidomide for multiple myeloma, 2–4 mg PO daily
Ponatinib	Tyrosine kinase inhibitor for ALL, CML
Posoconazole	Antifungal for candida, aspergilus, blastomycosis, mucormycosis, fusarium; 200 mg TID PO/300 mg IV daily
Piroxicam	NSAID, 10/20 mg cap; also gel
Pralatrexate	Related to methotrexate, used for lymphoma/leukemia
Pramipexole	Dopamine agonist for Parkinson's disease, restless leg syndrome; 0.25–1 mg TID
Pramlintide	Antidiabetic, amylin analog, 15–60 μg before each meal
Prasterone	Estrogen for vaginal application is post-menopause
Prasugrel	ADP receptor antagonist, antiplatelet for CAD; 5–10 mg PO OD
Pravastatin	Statin for dyslipidemia, 40–80 mg daily
Praziquantel	Pyrazine isoquinoline derivative for cysticercosis, echinococcosis, schistosomiasis; 20 mg/kg 6 hourly or 60 mg/kg single dose
Prazosin	Alfa 2, adreno receptor blocker for hypertension, 2.5/5 mg tab; 1–2 tab daily
Prednisolone/-Prednisone	Corticosteroid, for allergy, shock, asthma, arthritis, ALD, MS, serum sickness, 5, 10, 20, 40 mg tab; 10–20 mg of start, up to 60 mg daily
Pregabalin	Anticonvulsant, also for neuralgia, anxiety, restless leg, 75 mg cap/OD
Prednicarbate	Topical steroid
Pregnenolone	Intermediary in cortisone synthesis
Prenoxdiazine	Cough suppressant, 100 mg TID
Pretalvir	Helicase primase inhibitor, for HSV, VZV

Primaquine	Antimalarial for radical treatment, also useful in PCP; 7.5/15 mg tab; 15 mg daily × 14 days
Primidone	Anticonvulsant, 750–1000 mg/day
Probenecid	Given with penicillin and oseltamivir to raise their blood level by decreasing renal excretion; 500 mg tab 1 tab BID
Pritelivir	Helicase–primase inhibitor, antiviral like amenamevir for HSV, HZV
Procainamide	Antiarrhythmic for VT, PSVT; 15 mg/kg IV over 60 min
Procalcitonin	Inflammatory marker
Procarbazine	Alkylating agent, 50 mg cap; for lymphomas 100 mg/m^2 daily
Prochlor-perazine	Anti-emetic, also used in migraine, scombroid poisoning, 5 mg tab; 12.5 mg/ml inj.
Progesterone	100, 200, 400 mg tab, for progesterone deficiency; 200 mg HS
Proguanil	For malaria prophylaxis, 100 mg tab, 200 mg daily
Prolactin	Pineal hormone, helps in milk secretion
Promethazine	Antihistamine; 25 mg PO BID, IM/IV
Propafenone	Antiarrhythmic; 150–300 mg PO TID
Propofol	General anesthetic, also for delirium; 0.5–2 mg/hour infusion
Pegamidase	Enzyme to treat SCID
Proparacaine	For corneal anaesthesia, eye drop
Propoxyphene	Related to methadone, pain killer; 120 mg of it equivelant to 60 mg codein
Propranolol	Beta blocker for HTN, ataxia-tremor, movement disorder, CHD, thyrotoxicosis, postcoital headache, 80–120 mg BID
Propyl thiouracil	Anti-thyroid drug, 50 mg tab; 300–600 mg daily

Prostaglandin	For dysmenorrhea, pain, gastric mucosal defence
Prostaglandin E	For sunburn erythema
Prostaglandin-analogue	For glaucoma, peptic ulcer
Protamine	Heparin antagonist, 50 mg/5 ml inj; 1 mg neutralizes 50 units heparin
Prothionamide	Antitubercular, 25 mg/kg max. 2 g PO, OD
Protriptyline	Tricyclic antidepressant, helpful in cataplexy; 20–40 mg daily
Prucolapride	SHT4 agonist for constipation, 2 mg bed time
Psillicem	Bulk purgative
Pyrantel	For enterobiosis, ascariasis, trichinosis, 10 mg/kg, single dose
Pyrazinamide	Anti-tubercular, 500, 750 mg tab; 20 mg/kg daily
Pyridostigmine	For myasthenia gravis, 100–300 mg daily; also for orthostatic hypotension
Pyridoxine	For neurapathy, homocystinuria, INH toxicity, alcohol induced acidosis
Pyrimethamine	For malaria, toxoplasmosis, PCP prophylaxis, 50 mg daily incombination with sulfadoxin
Pyronaridine	Benzonaphthyridine antimalarial, more potent than chloroquine
Primidone	Antiepileptic, useful in ataxia and tremor, 50–250 mg PO daily
Propofol	Inhaled general anesthetic
Pyritinol	Cerebral function enhancer; 100–200 mg TID

Q

Qinghaosu	Artemisinin, the antimalarial agent
Quetiapine	For psychosis, bipolar disorder; 350–800 mg/day
Quinacrine	Used for giardiasis and SLE
Quinapril	5/10 mg tab; adjunct to diuretic and digoxin in CHF
Quinidine	Potent antimalarial; antiarrhythmic; 6–10 mg/kg IV/300–600 mg PO 6 hourly
Quinine	Anti malarial and also for babesiosis, 100/300 mg tab; 300–600 mg TID
Quinolines	Antibiotic group, DNA RNA synthesis inhibitors, e.g. ciprofloxacin, gemifloxacin, moxifloxacin, delafloxacin
Quinupristin–dalfopristin	Streptogramin group of antibiotic for MRSA 7.5 mg/kg IV 8 hourly

R

Racecadotril	For acute diarrhea; 100 mg cap TID
Rabeprazole	PPI for acid–peptic disease, 20 mg OD PO/IV
Raloxifene	Estrogen receptor modulator for gynaecomastia, breast cancer prevention and osteoporosis prevention, 60 mg/OD
Raltegravir	Anti-retroviral, 400 mg BID PO
Ramelteon	Melatonin receptor agonist for delirium
Ramipril	ACE inhibitor for HTN, CCF; 2.5–20 mg OD/QID
Ramosetron	$5HT_3$ antagonist, for vomiting of chemotherapy; 0.1 mg tab, 0.3 mg/day
Ramucirumab	VEGF antagonist for macular degeneration, cancer colon, lung, stomach
Ranitidine	PPI for peptic ulcer, 300 mg OD, also inj.
Ranibizumab	10 mg/ml inj. Intravitreal, for macular edema, AMD
Ranolazine	PPI for peptic ulcer, 300 mg OD
Rapamysin	Cardiac Na^+ current modulator for angina; 500 mg tab, 1 BID
Rapamysin	(Syn–Sirolimus)
Rasalazine	MAO B inhibitor, for Parkinsonism, 1 mg OD
Rasburicase	For uric acid nephropathy;
Reboxetine	Antidepressant, 2, 4 mg tab; 4 mg BID
Rasalagine	For Parkinson's disease; 0.5–1 mg daily
Regorafenib	Multikinase inhibitor for colon cancer, HCC, GIST
Renzapride	$5HT_4$ agonist, like cisapride
Repaglinide	Antidiabetic agent; 0.5–1 mg TID

Reserpine	Central sympatholytic for hypertension, 0.1 mg TID (with hydrochlorothazide 10 mg)
Remdesvir	For Covid-19; 200 mg IV day 1, then 100 mg IV for 4 days
Resveratrol	SIRTI agonist polyphenol, improves cardio-metabolic function
Reteplase	Recombinant tPA for thrombolysis, 2; 10 units bolus IV 30 min apart
Reviparin	AntiXa, prevention of thromboembolism, 0.6 ml PF syringe
Ribavirin	Antiviral for HCC, RSV; 15–25 mg/kg/day in 3 divided doses, oral, inhalation
Ribocicib	CDK4/6 inhibitor for metastatic breast cancer
Riboflavin	Vit B2 deficiency causes magenta tongue, angular stomatitis, corneal vascularization; 2 mg tab
Ravolizumab	MAB for PNH, HUS
Raxibacumab	For inhaled *B. anthracic* spores
Rifabutin, Rifampin, Rifapentine	Anti-tubercular agent, for prophylaxis and treatment, non tubercular mycobacteria, *H. pyori* eradication, gut sterilization in liver failure, Q fever, *H. influenzea* prophylaxis, anthrax, brucella, gas gangrene, leprosy, IBS, dose 10 mg/kg, maximum 600 mg OD
Rifaximin	For travellir's diarrhaea, hepatic coma, 200 mg TID for 3 days
Rilonacept	IL–I receptor fusion protein for familial Mediterrenean fever
Rilpivirine	Non nucleoside RTI for HIV, 25 mg QID
Riluzole	Glutamate transmission inhibitor for ALS
Rimantadine	Antiviral for influenza, 100 mg BID PO for 5–7 days
Riociguat	Soluble guanylyl cyclase stimulator for pulmonary hypertension, 2.5 mg PO TID

Risedronate	For osteoporosis and fracture prevention, 30 mg PO daily
Risperidone	For schizophrenia, bipolar disorder, 2–8 mg/day
Ritodrine	Anti HIV; 600 mg BID PO
Rituximab	Anti CD 20, for ALL, CLL, lymphoma, IgG4 disease, myasthenia, pemphigus, SLE, rheumatoid arthritis; 100 mg IV on day 0, 14
Rivaroxaban	Oral factor Xa inhibitor, anticoagulant; 10 mg start PO to 15 mg BID (for DVT, PE)
Rivastigmine	Used for Aizheimer disease 1.5, 3, 4, 5, 6 mg capsule
Rizatriptan	For migraine, 5 mg tab, maximum 30 mg/day
Rocuronium	Muscle relaxant, non depolarising
Rofecoxib	NSAID, cox inhibitor
Roflumilast	PDE4 inhibitor for COPD, chronic bronchitis, asthma like cilomilast, tofimilast
Romidepsin	HDAC inhibitor for T cell lymphoma
Romiplostim	TPO receptor agonist for ITP
Romosozumab	Humanized antibody decreasing scherostin, prevents osteoporosis; under evaluation
Ropinirole	Dopamine agonist for parkinsonism, 6–24 mg daily
Rosiglitazone	Anti-diabetic agent, a thiazolidinedione; 2, 4, 5 mg tab
Rosuvastatin	Statin for hyperlipidemia, 10 mg OD
Rotigotine	Dopamine agonist for Parkinsonism; patch 6–24 mg/day
Ropivacaine	7.5 mg/ml inj; local/regional anaesthesia
Roxatidine	PPI, 75 mg tab, and 150 mg forte tab
Ruxolitinib	Nonspecific JAK_2 inhibitor for polycythemia vera
Rufinamide	Antiepileptic, 45 mg/kg/day
Rupatadin	Anti-allergic, 10 mg tab OD

S

Sacubitril	Neprilysin inhibitor for heart failure, 100–200 mg BID
Safinamide	MAO B inhibitor for Parkinsonism, 100 mg OD
Salicylates	For rheumatic fever, SLE, antipyretic
Salbutamol	Bronchodilator for asthma, COPD, inhaler, 2 mg/4 mg tab;
Salicylic acid	Keratolytic for acne, tinea versicolor, warts
Samarium	For bone metastasis; 1 mCi/kg IV single dose
Salmeterol	Betaadrenergic agonist, bronchodilator; 50 μgm rotacap, 25 mcg metered dose inhaler
Salsalate	Oral NSAID and COX-2 inhibitor, analgesic; 1500 mg BID
Saquinavir	Protease inhibitor for HIV, 200/500 mg tab; 1000 mg BID
Sargramostim (GM–CSF)	For neutropenia of chemotherapy; 250 μg/kg/day
Saxagliptin	DPP4 inhibitor for DM_2, 2.5–5 mg OD/BID
Saroglitazar	Antidiabetic; 4 mg OD/BID
Scopolamine	Anticholinergic for vertigo, vomiting; transdermal patch
Secukinumab	Anti IL–17 A monoclonal for ankylosing spondylitis and psoriatic arthritis; 150 mg SC weekly
Secnidazole	For trichomoniasis, bacterial vaginosis, 2 g single dose
Selegiline	MAO-B inhibitor for Parkinsonism, depression; 5 mg BID, transdermal 6–12 mg/day
Selenium sulfide	Lotion for tinea versicolor

Selumetinib	For plexiform neurofibroma
Semaglutide	Long-acting GLP agonist for diabetes; 3, 7, 14 mg tab
Selexipag	Selective IP receptor agonist for pulmonary HTN
Sereloxin	For CHF, 30 μg/kg/min
Sertaline	Anti-depressant, 50–200 mg/day
Sevelamer	Phosphate binder, 400–800 mg tab
Sildenafil	Phosphodiesterage inhibitor, vasodilator for erectile dysfunction; 50/100 mg tab
Seratio peptidase	Anti-inflammatory enzyme, reduces edema, 5–15 mg TID; PAH, Rayaud's, CHF; 25–100 mg OD
Sibutramine	Appetite suppressant; 10 mg OD
Silibinin	Drug for hepatotoxic mushroom poisoning
Silodosin	For BPH, 4 mg/8 mg tab OD
Silver sulfa-diazine	Antiseptic–antibacterial, burn dressing
Simeprevir	Protease inhibitor for HCV genotype I, 4; 150 mg QID PO
Simethicone	Antiflatulant
Simvastatin	Statin for dyslipidemia, 20–80 mg daily
Silymarin	Hepatic protective, cholagogue; 140 mg BID/TID
Sisomycin	Aminoglycoside, local acting
Simethicone	Antiflatulant, 20–40 mg TID
Sirolimus	(Rapamycin)–immunosuppressant, stent life span enhancement, Kaposi sarcoma; 1 mg tab; 6 mg loading then 2 mg daily
Sitagliptin	DPP4 inhibitor for DM2, 50–100 mg daily
Sodium docusate	Purgative, 100 mg tab; up to 3 tab bedtime
Sodium fusidate	For bacterial skin infections, 2% ointment

Sodium-picosulphate	Purgative, 10 mg tab bedtime/liquid
Sodium-stibogluconate	Pentavalent antimonial for leishmaniasis
Sodium-sulfacetamide	For trachoma, local instillation, 10%, 20%
Sodium valproate	Antiepileptic, also used for bipolar disorder, migraine prevention, myoclonus, dyskinesia; 200/500 mg tab; chrono 250/300/500 mg tab; 600 mg daily
Sofosovir	Antiviral for HCV genotype 1, 4, 5, 6; dose 400 mg QID
Solifenacin	Agent for bladder dysfunction, urgency; 5–10 mg bedtime
Somatostatin	Haemostyptic; 250 mg bolus; ther 3.5 μg/kg 1 hour infusion
Somatropin	Growth hormone; 6–12 μg/kg/day; inshort stature, Turner syndrome, HIV wasting, short bowel syndrome, SHOX deficiency
Sonidegib	SMO inhibitor like vismodegib for basal cell carcinoma
Sorafenib	VEGFR pathway inhibitor for HCC and RCC; 400 mg PO BID
Sorbitol	Constiuent of hepatoprotectives
Sparfloxacin	Repiratory, soft tissue infection; 100/200 mg tab; 200–400 mg daily
Sotalol	Cardioselective beta blocker for hypertension; 80–160 mg BID
Spectinomycin	For gonococcal infection; 2 g IM QID
Spermidine	Enhances life and benefits neurodegeneration
Spiramycin	Used in toxoplasmosis, 3 MU tab; 6–9 MU daily
Spironolactone	Aldosterone antagonist for HTN, CHF, PCOD; 50 mg tab, 1–4/day

Sparfloxacin	Respiratory, soft tissue infection; 100/200 mg tab; 200–400 mg daily
Stanozolol	Anabolic steroid; 2 mg tab, 1–2 tab TID
Stavudine	Anti HIV, 30/40 mg cap BID
Streptokinase	Plasminogen activator for thrombolysis, 75,000–15,00,000 units
Streptomycin	Aminoglycoside antibiotic for tuberculosis, brucella; plague 1 g IM OD
Streptozotocin	Glucosamine nitrourea compound for neuroendocrine tumors
Strontium renelate	For osteoporosis; 4 mci IV every 2 months
Succimer (DMSA)	Indicated for lead poisoning
Succinyl choline	Depolarizing neuroparalysing agent often causing hyperkalemia
Sufentanyl	A fentayl congener, hypnotic; adjunct to general anaesthesia, 50 μg/ml/inj; muscle relaxant
Sucralfate	Gastric mucosal protective agent, 1 g QID
Sulbactam	Betalactamase inhibitor, also effective for *A. baumannii*; inj. 250/500 mg combined with ampicillin, ceftriaxone, cefotaxime
Sulfacetamide	Local agent for trachoma, 10%, 20% eye drop
Sulfadiazine	Antibacterial, by inhibiting dihydropteroate synthetase, useful in toxoplasmosis, Whipple disease; 500–1000 mg BID
Sulfadoxine	Anti malarial, 500 mg along with pyrimethamine 25 mg; 2–3 tab; single dose
Sulfa methoxazole	Dihydropteroate synthetase inhibitor and bacteriostatic; 800 mg given along with trimethoprim 160 mg
Sulfasalazine	Effective in ankylosing spondylitis, IBD, psoriatic arthritris, rheumatoid and reactive arthritis; dose– 500 mg PO BID

Sulfisoxazole	Sulfonamide like sulphmethoxazole
Sulphonyl urea	Anti-diabetic agents
Sulindac	NSAID, often causing cholestasis
Sumatriptan	$5HT_1$ agonist for migraine, cluster headache; 50–100 mg tab, 6 mg SC; nasal spray
Sunitinib	Typrosine kinase inhibitor for HCC, RCC, GIST; 50 mg daily PO
Suramin	Used for trypanosomiasis; 5 mg/kg IV day 1, then 20 mg/kg weekly
Suvorexant	Orexin receptor antagonist for insomnia, 10–20 mg tab

T

Tacrine	Cholinesterase inhibitor used for Alzheimer dementia; hepatotoxic
Tacrolimus	Immunosuppressant, for atopic dermatitis, SLE, myasthenia, post-transplant; 0.1–0.2 mg/kg/day in two divided doses
Tadalafil	PDE inhibitor for PAH, sexual dysfunction, Raynaud's phenomenon; 5–20 mg PO
Tafamidis	Agent for ATTR amyloidosis
Tafenaqine	8-aminoquinoline for malaria prophylaxis
Talazopasib	For myelodysplastic syndrome (PARP inhibitor) 1–1.5 g IV weekly
Tamoxifen	ER receptor modulator for breast cancer prophylaxis and prevention of osteoporosis, 20–40 mg/day
Tamsulosin	Alfa blocker for BPH, 0.2, 0.4 mg cap, 1–4 cap daily (often with dutasteride, finasteride)
Tasimeltion	Akin to remeltion, melatonin receptor agonist
Tapentadol	Pain killer, 50, 75, 100 mg tab, 50 mg 6 hourly
Targetrin	Retinoid for cutaneous T cell lymphoma
Tazarotene	Retinoid for topical therapy of psoriasis, acne
Tazobactom	Usually combined with piperacillin 4 g (4.5 g vial) for polymicrobial infection, IV infusion 8 hourly
Tecovirimat	Antiviral for monkey pox, 200 mg tab BID; 200 mg vial
Tedizolid	Oxazolidinediones, inhibit protein synthesis, effective for MRSA, Staph infection; 200 mg OD, PO/IV
Teduglutide	Recombinant GLP_2 for short bowel syndrome

Tegafur	Anti-cancer agent
Tegaserod	5HT4 agonist for IBS, now withdrawn
Teicoplanin	Glycopeptide antibiotic like vancomycin, 200–400 mg vial
Telaprevir	Protease inhibitor for HCV, 1st generation
Telavancin	Lipopeptide antibiotic for enterococci, streptococci, *S. aureus*
Telbivudine	Enantiomer of thyromidine for HBV; 600 mg/day PO
Telithromycin	Ketolide antibiotic for GM+ve organism; 800 mg PO OD
Telmisartan	Angiotensin II antagonist for HTN; 40–80 mg tab/OD
Telotristat	Tryptophan 5 hydroxylase inhibitor used in carcinoid syndrome
Temazepam	Anti-anxiety, insomnia; 15 mg PO
Temozolomide	Related to decarbazine, effective for CNS tumors, melanoma, ZES; 20, 100, 200 mg cap, 75 mg/m^2
Temsirolimus	mTOR inhibitor for RCC
Tenatoprazole	PPI with imidazopyridine ring, long acting
Tenectiplase	Recombinant tPA for fibrinolytic therapy in MI, stroke, PTE; 30–50 mg IV bolus
Teneligliptin	DPP4 inhibitor for DM2; 20 mg OD/BID
Tenoxicam	NSAID, 20 mg daily
Terconazole	5% vaginal cream and suppository for vulvovaginal candidiasis
Teniposide	For ALL, semisynthetic derivative of podophylotoxin
Tenofovir-disoproxil	Nucleotide analog for HBV, HIV; 300 mg/day PO
Tenofovir-alafenamide	Nucleotide analog for HBV, HIV; 25 mg/day PO

Terazosin	Alfa-adrenergic blocker for hypertension, neck spasm; 1–10 mg OD/BID
Terbinafine	Antifungal for tinea, onychomycosis, sporothrix; 250 mg OD to 500 mg BID PO
Terbutaline	Bronchodilator for bronchospasm; 2.5 mg tab TID
Terfenadine	Anti-allergic,100 mg PO BID; can cause QT prolongation
Teriflunomide	Agent for treatment of multiple sclerosis, 7–14 mg OD; inhibits orotate dehydrogenase
Teriparatide	1–34 PTH for osteoporosis, 250 μg inj.
Terizidone	Second line antitubercular agent
Terlipressin	Posterior pituitary hormone for hemostasis in bleeding peptic ulcer; 1 mg/ml 10 ml inj, 1–2 mg IV
Tesamorelin	For lipodystrophy caused by anti-HIV drugs
Testosterone	Cypionate, enanthate—male sex hormone, 40 mg cap, 1 cap TID
Tetrabenazine	Used for treatment of dystonia, tremor, chorea, 25 mg tab; ½ TID
Tetracycline	Bacterial protein synthesis inhibitor (30s ribosomal binding) for acne, actinomycosis, cholera; legionella, malaria, plague, syphilis, sprue; 250/500 mg cap, 1–2 g daily in 4 divided doses
Tetrathiomolybdate	Copper chelator for Wilson's disease
Thalidomide	Used in multiple myeloma, myelofibrosis, ankylosing spondylitis, Behcet's; 50–200 mg PO QID
Theophylline	Bronchodilator; tab, inj, syrup (along with etophylline)
Thiabendazole	For strongyloidiasis, cutaneous larva migrans

Thiazides	Diuretic for ascites, edema
Thiocolchi-coside	Muscle relaxant, 4 mg, 8 mg tab, also inj; 8 mg daily
Thiazolidine-diones	Promote glucose utilization, increase insulin synthesis, used in DM2–NAFL
Thienopyridines	Clopidogrel, prasugrel, ticlopidine
Thioguanine	Antimetabolite; for AML, ALL, 100 mg/m^2 PO BID on days 1–5; for cancer, ovary, breast, NHL, HD; 10–20 mg/m^2 IV every 4 weeks
Thimerisal	Agent causing contact dermatitis
Thiopental	General anesthetic
Thioridazine	Antipsychotic; 10–75 mg PO 8 hourly
Tibolone	2.5 mg tab, for menopausal symptoms, osteoporosis
Thiotepa	Cancer chemotherapy agent
Thyroxine	25, 50; 100 μg tab for hypothyroidism
Thiothixene	High potent antipsychotic
Tiagabine	Antiepileptic; 32–56 mg/day
Tianeptin	12.5 mg tab, for depression, 1 tab TID
Ticagrellor	P2 Y12 inhibitor, orally active anti-platelet drug for CAD; 130 mg loading, then 90 mg PO BID
Ticarcillin - Clavulanate	For anaerobes, broad spectrum antibiotic 3.1 g vial, 1 vial 6 hourly
Ticlopidine	ADP receptor blocker in platelets, given in TIA; 250 mg PO BID
Tigecycline	Bacterial protein synthesis inhibitor used in conditions akin to tetracycline; 100 mg IV loading, then 50 mg IV BID
Tiludronate	Bisphosphonate for osteoporosis, Paget's disease; 800 mg PO daily
Tetrathio-molybdate	Copper absorption prevention in Wilson's disease

Tiludronate	Bisphosphanate for Paget's disease, 800 mg PO daily
Timolol	Beta blocker for IHD, local eye drop for glaucoma; 10 mg BID; 0.25–0.5% eye drop twice daily
Tinidazole	Nitro imidazole effective for amoebiasis, giardiasis, trichomoniasis, 300–500 mg TID
Tinzaparin	Non warfarin anticoagulant for thrombo-embolism (PTE); 75 U/kg SC OD
Tiopronin	Cystine binder, used in cystinuria; 800–1200 mg PO daily
Tioconazole	Cream for vulvovaginal candidiasis
Tiotropium	Anticholinergic bronchodilator, used in asthma; 18 µg rotacap
Tirofiban	GP IIb/IIIa inhibitor for acute coronary syndrome; 25 µg/kg bolus, then 0.15 µg/kg/min infusion
Tivantinib	Drug for HCC; NET inhibitor like cobozatinib
Tivozamib	Drug for HCC; NET inhibitor like cobozatinib
Tizanidine	Alfa2 adrenergic agonist to treat muscle spasm, 2 mg tab, maximum 36 mg daily in divided doses
Tobramycin	Aminoglycoside for *E. coli*, pseudomonas, CAP; 0.3% eye drop
Tocilizumab	IL-6 receptor antibody for RA, arteritis and PSS, 4–8 mg/kg IV/month, also for Covid-19
Tocotrienol	Used for treatment of diseases due to mtDNA point mutation
Tofacitinib	JAK 1, JAK 3 inhibitor for RA, AS, IBD, psoriatic arthritis; 5 mg PO BID
Tolazamide	Sulphonyl urea, anti-diabetic; 900–1000 mg OD
Tolbutamide	Antidiabetic agent, 1–2 g daily as single dose

Tolcapone	COMT inhibitor for Parkinson's disease, 100–200 mg TID
Tolfenamic acid	NSAID for acute migraine; 200 mg PO
Tolnaftate	Antifungal ointment
Tolterodine	For bladder hperreflexia, 2 mg TID
Tolvaptan	AVP antagonist for SIADH, hypervolemic hyponatremia, 15–30 mg OD
Topiramate	Anti-convulsant, migraine prevention, 200–400 mg/day
Toremifene	Antiestrogen, 60 mg PO daily for breast cancer
Topotecan	Topoisomerase poison for lung, ovarian cancer, 1.5 mg/m^2 IV daily for 5 days every 3 weeks
Torsemide	Loop diuretic, 10–100 mg daily
Tositumomab	Monoclonal for NHL
Trabectedin	For sarcoma, 1 mg vial; 1.5 mg/m^2 IV infusion
Tramadol	For pain relief in neuropathy, 37.5 mg tab, BID/TID; 50–100 mg/inj.
Trametinib	MEK inhibitor for melanoma
Triamterene	K^+ retaining diuretic, 50–100 mg OD/BID
Trandolapril	ACE inhibitor for CHF; 0.5–4 mg OD
Tranexamic acid	Antifibrinolytic for capillary bleed (CNS), 500 mg PO TID; menorrhagia
Trastuzumab	HER_2 *neu* antibody for breast cancer, 4 mg/kg IV loading; then 2 mg/kg IV weekly
Travoprost	For glaucoma; 0.004%, 1 drop daily
Trazodone	For insomnia, post-traumatic stress disorder (PTSD); 150–375 mg/day
Tranylcy-promine	Antidepressant, 20–50 mg/day
Tremelimumab	Anti CTLA4 for HCC

Treprostinil	Prostacyline derivative for PAH, IV/SC/inhalation, oral
Tretinoin	For acne, mycosis fungoides, 45 mg/m^2 PO daily
Triamcinolone	Fluorinated glucocorticoid, mostly used locally
Triamterene	Potassium sparing diuretic for HTN, 50 mg tab, OD
Triclabendazole	Benz imidazole active against fasciolopsiasis and paragonimus species; 10 mg/kg once/twice PO
Triazolam	For anxiety, insomnia; 0.125, 0.250 mg tab
Triclophos	500 mg/5 ml, for insomnia
Trientine	Copper chelator for Wilson's disease; 250 mg cap, 1–1.5 g daily
Trifluperazine	1st generation anti-psychotic, 5 mg tab, 1 tab TID
Trifluperidol	Antipsychotic, 0.5 mg tab, OD
Trifluridine	Pirimidine nucleoside for HSV, CMV, topical therapy
Trihexyphenidol	Anticholinergic for dystonia, Parkinsonism, 2 mg tab, start 1 OD, increase up to 15 mg
Trilostane	11β-hydroxylase inhibitor, inhibits steroidogenesis in Cushing syndrome
Trimetazidine	For angina, 20 mg tab TID
Trimethoprim	Structural analog of pteridine, inhibits dihydrofolate reductase, bacteriostatic; used for *P. carinii* pneumonia, 5 mg/kg PO/IV along with SMX
Trimetrexate	Dihydrofolate reductase inhibitor akin to trimethoprim
Triptorelin - pamoate	GNRH analog; 3.75 mg IM every month

Troglitazone	PPRY agonist, insulin sensitizer for DM, now withdrawn, causes liver failure
Tropisetron	$5HT_3$ receptor antagonist for diarrhoea of carcinoid syndrome
Tropicamide	Mydriatic, 1%, for eye exm
Tumstatin	Angiogenesis inhibitor
Trimethoprim–Sulfa-methoxazole	Effective in staph, MRSA, brucellosis, pertussis, plague, PCP, legionella, listeria, brucella, CGD, melioidosis
Tripolidine	Antiallergic, 1.25 mg in combination
Tyrothricin	0.05% ear drop for external otitis

U

Ulipristal	Oral anti-progestin for postcoital contraception, 30 mg tab
Ubidecarenone	Supplement, cardiac adjuvant
UDCA	Cholagogue, cholelitholytic, hepatic protector, 75, 150, 300 mg tab, 8–10 mg/kg daily in 3 divided doses
Ularitide	Vasodilator for CHF, 15 mg/kg/min infusion
Umeclidinium	LAMA for bronchial asthma
Ustekinumab	Monoclonal AB to IL–23/IL 12 for psoriasis and psoriatic arthritis
Urokinase	Fibrinolytic, antiplatelet for thrombus dissolution, used in CAD; pulmonary embolism; 2 lac units bolus IV
Urofolitropin	(FSH) 75 IU amp, ovulation induction 75–150 IU daily
Ursodeoxycholic acid	For cholesterol rich gallstone dissolution; 300 mg TID

V

Vaborabactam	Beta lactamase inhibitor combined with meropenem for gram–negative sepsis
Valbenazine	$VMAT_2$ inhibitor for tardive dyskinesia
Valacyclovir	Antiviral for HSV, HZV, 500 mg, 1 g tab; 1 g TID
Valenthamate	Anticholinergic smooth muscle relaxant tab, 1 g TID
Valvenazine	Ester of tetrabenazine for tardive dyskinesia
Valdecoxib	Non-narcotic analgesic; 10–20 mg PO BID
Valganciclovir	Antiviral for CMV, 900 mg PO BID
Valproic acid	Antiepileptic, also for migraine, myoclonus, bipolar disorder, tardive dyskinesia, panic disorder, 20–60 mg/kg
Valomaciclovir	Antiviral for CMV, HSV; helicase primase inhibitor
Valrubicin	For uroepithelial cancer
Valsartan	Angiotensin II antagonist for HTN, 80 mg tab, OD
Vancomycin	Glycopeptide antibiotic for MRSA, endocarditis, TSS, necrotizing fasciitis, 15 mg/kg BID IV; 125 mg PO QID
Vandetanib	TKI for lung and thyroid cancer; RET, VEGFR, EGFR antagonist
Vapendavir	Antiviral for enteroviruses
Vardenafil	Phosphodiesterase inhibitor for erectile dysfuncion; 5–10 mg PO
Varenicline	Drug for smoking cessation, 0.5, 1 mg tab, maintenance dose 1 mg twice daily

Vasoactive intestinal–polypeptide	IV infusion for ARDS, 150 μg/10 ml daily × 3 days
Vecuronium	Depolarizing agent for anesthesia/intubation, 4 mg amp.
Vedolizumab	Anti-integrin for IBD
Velpatasvir	Antiviral for HCV, 100 mg OD
Verubecestar	For β amyloid reduction of Alzheimer disease
Vemurafenib	BRAF inhibitor for lung cancer, melanoma, hairy cell leukemia
Venlafaxine	Antidepressant, also for PTSD, panic attack, 75–375 mg/day
Venetoclax	BCL_2 inhibitor for CLL
Verapamil	Calcium channel blocker for HTN, angina, AF, cluster headache, SVT, CAD; 80–160 mg 8 hourly
Vidarabine	Purine nucleoside analog for HSV, HZV, EBV; topical 3% ointment
Vilazodone	Norepinephrine serotonin reuptake inhibitor for depression; 40 mg/day
Vildagliptin	DPP4 inhibitor for DM2; 50 mg OD
Vinblastine	Vinca alkaloid for bladder cancer; dose 0.1–0.2 mg/kg IV weekly
Vincristine	Mitotic spindle inhibitor for ALL, lung/breast cancer, Ewing sarcoma; 1.5 mg/m^2, maximum 2 mg weekly
Vinorelbine	Mitotic spindle inhibitor for ALL, lung/breast cancer, Ewing sarcoma; 25 mg/m^2 IV weekly
Vismodegib	Hedgehog pathway inhibitor for metastatic basal cell cancer
Voglibose	Alfaglucosidase inhibitor for DM2; 0.3 mg TID

Vorapaxar	PAR–I antagonist; anticoagulant for MI, stroke
Voriconazole	Anti-fungal for candida, aspergillus, trichosporum; 200 mg–400 mg PO, OD
Vorinostat	HDAL inhibitor for ALL, 200–400 mg IV OD
Vortioxetine	Serotonin and norepinephrine reuptake inhibitor for depressive disorder; 5–20 mg/day
Voxilaprevir	Antiviral for HCV
Volanesersen	APO CIII inhibitor to reduce triglycerides

W

Warfarin	Anticoagulant, antiplatelet, fibrinolytic; 10–15 mg PO daily

X

Xanthinol-nicotinate	150 mg tab, 300 mg cap, 500 mg retard, 1–2 tab twice daily; IV infusion maximum 950 mg daily
Ximelagatran	Direct oral thrombin inhibitor for stroke, thromboembolism
Xylometazoline	Nasal decongestant, nasal drop

Y

Yttrium	Beta emitter for radioembolization

Z

Zafirlukast	Leukotriene antagonist for asthma, 20 mg tab/BID
Zalcitabine	Nucleotide–nucleoside reverse transcription inhibitor for HIV
Zaleplon	Hypnotic sedative, 5, 10 mg cap, 10 mg HS
Zanamivir	Antiviral for influenza, 10 mg/day oral/inhalation
Zidovudine	Antiviral for HIV, adult T cell lymphoma/leukemia; 200 mg PO 8 hourly
Zileuton	Lox inhibitor for asthma (now, withdrawn)
Ziprasidone	Used for bipolar disorder, schizophrenia; 120–200 mg/day
Zirconium	Substance that produces red brown skin lesions like sarcoidosis, also used in gentamicin chained beads for implantation in chronic bone infection
Zoledronate	Bisphosphonate for osteoporosis, hypercalcemia; 4 mg IV every month
Zolmitriptan	Triptan for migraine; 5 mg nasal spray; 2.5 mg tab; maximum 10 mg/day
Zolpidem	Hypnotic–sedative; 5, 10 mg tab, 1 HS
Zonisamide	Anti-convulsant, 200–400 mg/day
Zotarolimus	Stent coating agent to prevent stent thrombosis
Zopiclone	Hypnotic–sedative, 7.5 mg tab 1 HS
Zotepine	Antipsychotic, 25 mg TID

Part II

Drugs of Last Decade

A

Abametapir	For head lice
Abemaciclib	For breast cancer
Abrocitinib	To treat atopic dermatitis
Acarbose	Alfa glucosidase inhibitor for DM_2
Acesulfane	Artificial sweetner
Acetylcystine	Mucolytic, oral/inhalation; 200 mg TID
Adagracib	To treat non-small cell lung cancer
Adrecizumab	Adrenomedullin antibody for septic shock
Aducanumab	No antibody for Alzheimer disease
Afamelanotide	For phototoxic skin reaction of erythropoietic protoporphyria
Alalerono-difloxacin	For Staph septicemia
Alfatoco	For Leish syndrome
Alirocumab	Lipid lowering agent
Alitretinoin	For AIDS related sarcoma
Alpelisib	P13k inhibitor for breast cancer
Amisulpiride	Schizophrenia, 400–800 mg daily, prevention of vomiting after surgery
Amivantamab	For NSC lung cancer
Anacaulase-bcdb	Escar removal of full thickness thermal burn
Anifrolumab	For SLE
Ansuvimab	To treat Ebola
Apalutamide	For prostate cancer
Aprenavir	Antiviral for HIV
Articaine	Long acting local anaesthetic
Asciminib	For pH +ve multiple myeloma

Aspertame	Artificial sweetner
Atogepant	For migraine prevention
Atosiben	Oxytocin antagonist for preterm labor
Avacopan	For granulomatosis with polyangitis
Avalogluco-sidase alfa	Pompe's disease
Avapritinib	For unresectable GI cancer
Avapritinib	For systemic mastocytosis
Avatrombopeg	For thrombocytopenia
Azelnidipine	For hypertension
Maftivimab, Odesivimab	To treat Ebola

B

Balaxavir	For influenza
Baricitinib	For rheumatoid arthritis
Belantamab mafodotin	For multiple myeloma
Belimosudil	For chronic graft-versus-host disease
Belzutifan	For von Hippel Lindau disease
Bempedoic acid	Lipid lowering agent
Benralizumab	Anti IL5 for asthma
Berotralstat	For hereditary angioedema
Bictegravir	Integrase inhibitor for HIV
Bimonidin	Anti-glaucoma agent
Binimetinib	For melanoma
Bremelanotide	For hyposexuality of premenopause
Brexanolone	For postpartum depression
Brolucizumab	VEGF inhibitor for macular degeneration
Burosumab	For X-linked hypophosphatemia

C

Canabidiol	For epilepsy
Canegermin	For keratitis
Caplacizumab	For acquired thrombotic thrombocytopenic purpura
Capmatinib	For NSC lung cancer
Casimersen	For Duchenne muscular dystrophy
Cedazuridine	For myelodysplastic syndrome
Cefiderocol	For resistant UTI
Cemiplimab	For squamous carcinoma
Cenobamate	For partial onset seizure, dose 125–200 mg/day
Ciprofibrate	Lipid lowering agent
Citacabtagene	IV for multiple myeloma
Clascoterone	For acne
Clodronate	For breast cancer
Colesevalam	Bile acid binding agents to reduce cholesterol
Colestipiol	Cholesterol lowering agent
Crizanlizumab	For sickle cell pain crisis
Cyclosilicate	For hyperkalemia
Cysteamine bitartarate	For mt DNA disorders

D

Dacomitinib	For NSC lung cancer
Daridorexant	JAK-1 inhibitor for insomnia
Darolutamide	For non-metastatic prostate cancer
Daxibotuli-numtoxinA	To treat glabellar line
Decitabine - cedazuridine	Adult MDS
Deucravacitinib	To treat plaque psoriasis
Dextroam-phetamine transdermal	For ADHD
Difelikefalin	For pruritus of CKD
Doravirine	For HIV
Dostarlimab	For endometrial cancer
Droperidol	Antipsychotic agent
Drospireone	For contraception
Dupilumab	Anti IL-4 for asthma

E

Efgartigimod	For myasthenia gravis
Eflapegrastim	To treat febrile neutropenia after myelosuppressive therapy
Elagolix	For pain of endometriosis
Elamipritide	For mt DNA disorders
Elexacaftor, tezacaftor	For cystic fibrosis
Eloctate	Factor VIII Fc conjugate for hemophilia
Endoxaban	Direct acting oral anticoagulant
Endoxifan	For acute mania
Enfortumab	For bladder cancer
Enfuviritide	Fusion inhibitor for HIV
Entrectinib	For metastatic bladder cancer
Ephedrine	Sympathomimetic for nasal congestion, hypotension
Epitnezumab	For migraine prevention
Eravacycline	Abdominal sepsis
Erenumab	For migraine
Ertugliflozin	$SGLT_2$ inhibitor for DM_2
Evinacumab	For familial hypercholesterolemia

F

Faricimab	Intravitrial for macular edema, degeneration
Fenspiride	For rhinosinusitis
Fexinidazole	For trypanosomiasis
Finerenone	For CKD of DM
Flortacipir F18	Diagnostic agent for multiple sclerosis
Fostamatinib	For immune thrombocytopenia, myelofibrosis
Fostemsavir	For HIV
Fremanezumab	Antimigraine
Futibatinib	To treat intrahepatic cholangiocarcinoma

G

Gadopiclenol	MRI contrast
Galcanezumab	Migraine prophylaxis
Ganaxolone	For seizure of cyclin dependent kinase like 5 deficiency
Ganaxolone	For status epilepticus
Givosiran	For hepatic porphyria
Glecaprevir	Protease inhibitor for HIV
Golodirsen	For Duchhene muscular dystrophy

I

Ibalizumab	For multi-drug resistant HIV
Ibrexafungerp	For vulvo vaginal candidiasis
Idelvion	Factor IX albumin conjugate for haemophila
Iguratimod	For rheumatoid arthritis
Inclisiran	For familial hypercholesterolemia
Inebilizumab	For neuromyelitis optica
Infigratinib	For cholangiocarcinoma
Iofexitin	For opium withdrawal
Ipragliflozin	$SGLT_2$ inhibitor for DM_2
Isatuximab	For multiple myeloma
Istradefylline	For on–off feature of Parkinsonism
Ivacaftor–tezacaftor	For cystic fibrosis

L

Lanadelumab	For hereditary angioedema
Lasimiditan	For migraine
Lefamulin	For community acquired pneumonia
Lemborexant	For insomnia
Lenacapavir	For resistant HIV infection
Levomil-ansipran	For depression
Libervant	For acute repetitive seizure
Lonafarnib	For premature aging
Lonapeg - somatropin	For short stature
Loncastuximab	For large B cell lymphoma
Loriatinib	For NSC lung cancer
Lorlatinib	For lymphoma
Lumasiran	For hyperoxaluria type 1
Lumatepe-rone tosylate	For schizophrenia
Lurbinectedin	For metastatic small cell lung cancer
Luspatercept	Used in beta thalassemia, to reduce transfusion requirement
Lusutrombopeg	For thrombocytopenia
Lutetium dotatate	For neuroendocrine, gastropancreatic cancer

M

Maralixibat	For pruritus of cholestasis
Margetuximab	For HER (2) positive breast cancer
Maribavir	For CMV (Post-transplant)
Mavacamten	To treat obstructive hypertrophic cardio-myopathy
Melphalan–flufenamide	For refractory multiple myeloma
Migalastat	For Fabry's disease
Mirabegran	For over active bladder
Mirvetuximab	To treat resistant ovarian cancer
Mitapivat	For pyruvate kinase deficient hemolytic anemia
Mobocertinib	For NSC lung cancer
Mogamulizumab	For NHL
Mosunetuzumab	To treat non Hodgkin's lymphoma
Moxdectin	For onchocerciasis

N

Naxitamab	For neuroblastoma
Nifurtimox	For Chagas disease
Nivolumab	PD_1 blocking antibody for melanoma

O

Odevixibat	For severe pruritus
Odimertumab	For colon cancer
Oliceridin	For pain management
Olipudase alfa	To treat sphingomyelinase deficiency
Olutasidenib	To treat refractory AML
Omaveloxolone	For mt DNA disorders
Omidenepag	For ocular hypertension, open angle glaucoma
Opicapon	For on–off periods of Parkinsonism
Osilodrostat	For Cushing syndrome, with failed pituitary surgery
Oteseconazole	For vulvovaginal candidiasis
Ozanimod	For multiple sclerosis, relapse

P

Pacritinib	For myelofibrosis with thrombocytopenia
Pacritinib	To treat myelofibrosis
Pafolacianine	For ovarian cancer detection
Patisiran	For polyneuropathy of amyloidosis
Pegaptanib	VEGF inhibitor for macular degeneration
Pegcetacoplan	For paroxysmal nocturnal haemoglobinuria
Pegvalinase	For phenylketonuria
Pemigatinib	For cholangio carcinoma
Pexidartinib	For tenosynovial giant cell lymphoma
Pitolisant	For adult narcolepsy
Pixantrone	For NHL
Plazomicin	For UTI
Ponesimod	For relapsing multiple sclerosis
Prabotulinum-toxin	For facial cosmesis akin to botulinom toxin
Pralsetinib	For NSC lung cancer
Pretomanid	For pulmonary tuberculosis

R

Relugolix	For advanced prostate cancer
Remdesvir	For Covid-19
Remimazolam	For anxiety, insomnia
Revefenacin	For COPD
Rimegrepant	For migraine
Ripasudil eye drop	For glaucoma
Ripretinib	For advanced gastrointestinal stromal tumor
Risankitumab	For plaque psoriasis
Risdiplam	For spinal muscular atrophy
Romosozumab	For post-menopausal osteoporosis
Ropeginter-feron–alfa 2b	For polycythemia vera

S

Sacituzumab - govitecan	For triple, negative breast cancer
Safinamide	For Parkinsonism
Samidorphen	For schizophrenia
Sarecycline	For NSLC
Satralizumab	For neuromyelitis optica
Segesteron	Vaginal ring for contraception
Selinexor	For refractory multiple myeloma
Selpercatinib	For lung and thyroid cancer
Selumetinib	For neurofibromatosis type I
Serdexmethyl-phenidate	For ADHD
Setmelanotide	For obesity of promelanocortin deficiency
Sinecatachin	For local application on warts
Siponimod	For multiple sclerosis
Sofinamide	For Parkinsonism
Solriamfetol	For hypersomnia of adults
Somapacitan	Growth hormone
Sotorasib	NSC lung cancer
Spesolimab	For generalized pustular psoriasis flares
Sutimlomab	For cold agglutinin disease

T

Tafacitamab	For large B cell lymphoma
Tafamidis - meglumine	For cardiomyopathy of amyloidosis
Tafenaquine	For malaria
Tanapanor	For IBS
Tapinarof	To treat plaque psoriasis
Tazametostat	For epitheloid sarcoma
Tazemetostat	IGF-1 inhibitor for follicular lymphoma, epithelioid sarcoma
Tebentafusp	For uveal melanoma
Teclistamab	For refractory multiple myeloma
Telotristat	Serotonin synthesis inhibitor for carcinoid syndrome
Tenapanor	For irritable bowel syndrome
Teplizumab	To delay progression of type 1 diabetes mellitus
Tepotinib	For non-small cell lung cancer
Teprotumumab	For thyroid eye disease
Tezacaftor, Ivacaftor	For cystic fibrosis
Tezepelumab	For asthma maintenance
Tildrakizumab	For plaque psoriasis
Tirbanibulin	For actinic keratosis of face and scalp
Tirzepatide	To improve blood sugar profile in diabetics
Tisotimab vidontin	For metastatic cancer cervix
Tralokinumab	For atopic dermatitis
Tremelimumab	For unresectable hepatocellular cancer

Triclabendazole	For fasciolopsiasis
Trifarotene	Topical application in acne vulgaris
Triheptanoin	For long chain fatty acid oxidation disorders
Trilaciclib	For chemotherapy induced myelosuppression
Tucatinib	For HER_2 positive breast cancer

U

Ubrogepant	For migraine
Umbralisib	For follicular lymphoma
Upadacitinib	For moderately severe rheumatoid arthritis

V

Venolizumab	For neuropathic pain
Vericiguat	For CHF with reduced ejection fraction
Vibegron	To treat overactive bladder
Viloxazine	For attention deficit hyperactivity disorder
Vitolarsen	For Duchenne muscular dystrophy
Voclosporin	Calcineurin inhibitor for lupus nephritis
Vonoprazan	For combination therapy of *H. pylori* with amoxicillin, clarithromycin
Vosoritide	For achondroplasia
Voxelotor	For sickle cell disease
Vutrisiran	For polyneuropathy of amyloidosis

Z

Zanubrutinib	For mantle cell lymphoma

Part III

Glimpses from Pharmacology

Drugs and Diseases

ADP blockers: Clopidogrel, Prasugrel, Ticlopidine

Platelet maturation inhibitor—anagrelide

PAR-I inhibitors—atoxapar, vorapaxar

Drugs Causing Thrombocytopenia

Acetazolamide, aspirin, carbamazepine, carbenicillin Chlorpropamide, chlorthalidone, clotrimazole, digoxin Furosemide, gold, heparin, indomethacin, INH, methyldopa, oxyphenbutazone, phenytoin, quinidine, quinine, thiazides, ticarcillin

Penicillin (Derived from Penicillicum Chrysogenum) Drug of Choice for

Syphilis, actinomycosis, gas gangrene, anaerobic infections leptospirosis, viridans streptococci (group A and B)

Yaws, rat bite fever

Ureidopenicillins—azlocillin, mezlocillin, piperacillin

Ceftriaxone is drug of choice for enteric fever, gonorrhea
E.coli, Proteus, Haemophillus, Serratia

For pseudomonas, DOC are:
Ceftazidime, cefepirome, cefepime
Cefoperazone, moxalactam

For anaerobes; DOC—vancomycin, metronidazole, clindamycin
Fluoroquinolone (4th generation)

Streptogramins like quinipristin and dalfopristin
are only needed for MRSA, VRSA, LRSA
resistant pneumococci

4th generation Quinolones are moxifloxacin, ferofloxacin
garenofloxacin, gemifloxacin

Antipsychotics

Typical

Aliphatic – chlorpromazine, proclorperazine, triflupromazine
Piperazines – flufenazine, trifluperazine
Piperidines – mesoridazine, thioridazine
Butyrophenones – droperidol, haloperidol
Miscellaneous – amisulpiride, molindone, pimozide, sulpiride

Atypical

Clozapine, aripiprazole, olanzapine, quetiapine
Iloperidone, paliperidone, risperidone
Sertindole, ziprasidone
Others—asenapine, lusaridone

Drugs for IBS

Diarrhoea predominant	*Constipation–predominant*
Alosetron, mebeverine	Linaclotide
Fedozotine, clonidine	Loxiglutide
Loperamide darifenacin	Lubiprostone
Solifenacin	Tegaserod

Direct Thrombin Inhibitors

Oral – dabigatran
Parenteral – Argatroban, bivaluridin, hirudin, lepirudin

Factor Xa Inhibitors

Oral—apixaban, rivaroxaban
Parenteral—argotroban, enoxaparin, daltroban, sultroban
Glycoprotein IIb/IIIa inhibitors—eptifibatide

Malaria Treatment

1. *P. vivax, P. ovale, P. malariae*
   CQ 10 mg/kg, then 5 mg/kg after 6 hours, then 25 mg/kg for next 2 days (total 25 mg/kg) + primaquine 15 mg daily × 14 days
2. If CQ resistant
   Quinine 10 mg/kg TID × 7 days + doxycycline 100 mg daily × 7 days or clindamycin 600 mg BID × 7 days + primaquine as above
3. CQ resistance (usually *P. falciparum*)
   a. Artesunate 4 mg/kg/day × 3 days + sulfadoxine 500 mg/pyrimethamine 75 mg single dose
   b. Artesunate as above + mefloquine 15 mg/kg × 3 days
   c. Artemether 80 mg + lumefantrine 480 mg twice daily × 3 days
   d. Arterolane 150 mg + piperaquine 750 mg daily × 3 days
   e. Quinine 600 mg TID × 7 days + doxycycline 100 mg OD or Clindamycin 600 mg BID × 7 days
4. Complicated malaria
   a. Artesunate 2–4 mg/kg IV/IM, repeat after 12, 24 hours then OD × 7 days
   b. Arteether 3.2 mg/kg IM then 1.6 mg/kg IM daily × 7 days
   c. Artemether as above
   d. Quinine 20 mg/kg IV in 5D St then 15 mg/kg in dextrose saline, switch over to oral quinine 10 mg/kg 8 hourly to complete 7 days of therapy

Toxicity of Quinolones

Gatifloxacin, sparfloxacin	hypo-/hyperglycemia
Trovafloxacin	hepatotoxic
Temafloxacin	haemolysis
Sparfloxacin	QT prolongation
Lomefloxacin, sparfloxacin	phototoxicity

Antibiotics; Mechanism of Action

Cellwall inhibition—beta lactams, bacitracin, vancomycin

Protein synthesis inhibition—macrolides, tetracyclines, aminoglycosides, linezolid, dalfopristin, quinopristine, tetracyclines

Cell membrane—gramicidin, polymyxin

DNA synthesis inhibitor—quinolones, novobiocin

Nucleic acid synthesis inhibition—rifampicin, nitrofurantoin, metronidazole

Uses of Nitroimidazole (Metronidazole)

Amoebiasis, anaerobic infections, bacterial vaginosis

H. pylori, vincents infections, Ludwig angina, giardiasis

Antifungals

Cellwall inhibitors—eichinocandins, nikkomycins (anidulafungin, caspofungin)

Cell membrane inhibitors—azoles, amphotericin B, terbinafine

DNA damage—flucytosine

Microtubules inhibitors—griseofulvin

Azoles include fluconazole, ketoconazole, itraconazole, posoconazole voriconazole

Antimalarials

Prophylaxis	– Chloroquine, mefloquine, proguanil
Radical cure	– Primaquine, tafenaquine
Clinical cure	– Chloroquine, mefloquine, amodiaquine, lumefantrine, halofantrine, atovaquone, quinine, artemisinins

Chemical Classification of Antimalarials

1. 4-Aminoquinolines—amodiaquine, chloroquine, piperaquine, mepacrine and quinacrine
2. 8-Aminoquinolines—bulaquine, primaquine, tafenaquine

3. Cinchona alkaloids—quinine sulphate
4. Biguanides—cycloguanil, proguanil
5. Sesquiterpine lactone—mefloquine
6. Napthoquinone—atovaquone, pyronaridine, naphthyridine
7. Phenanthrenes—halofantrine, lumefantrine
8. Artemisinins—arteether, artemether, artesunate, arterolane, dihydroartemisinin
9. Sulfonamides—sulfadoxine + pyrimethamine
   Sulfamethopyrazine
   Dapsone
10. Antibiotics—clindamycin, doxycycline, tetracycline

Antitubercular Drugs

1st line: INH, rifampicin, ethambutol, pyrazinamide, streptomycin, thiacetazone, rifabutin, rifapentine

2nd line: Ethionamide, prothionamide, cycloserine, kanamycin, capreomycin

3rd line: For MDR TB—Bedaquiline, delamanid

Anti-HIV Drugs

NRTI—Zidovudine, lamivudine, stavudine, didanosine; zalcitabine, abacavir

NNRTI—Efavirenz, nevirapine, delavirdine, etravirine, rilpivirine

Nucleotide RTI—tenofovir

Protease inhibitors—ritonavir, azatanavir, indinavir, tipranavir, darunavir

Fusion inhibitors—enfuvirtide

Entry inhibitors—maraviroc, vicriviroc

Intigrase inhibitors—dolutegravir, elvitagravir, raltegravir

Maturation inhibitor—bevirimat

Others—Cobicistat

Drugs for Chronic Hepatitis B

- Interferon
- Lamivudine, telbivudine, tenofovir
- Emtricitabine

Chronic HDV

- Interferons, lonafarnib

Chronic HCV

- Interferons, ribavirin
- Protease inhibitors

Simeprevir, sofosbuvir, ledipasvir, elbasvir paritaprevir, ritonavir dasabuvir, ombitasvir, daclatasvir, grazoprevir, ombitasvir velpatasvir, grazoprevir, saquinavir

Monoclonal Antibodies, Indications

Cetuximab	Colon cancer, squamous carcinoma head and neck
Rituximab	Lymphoma, leukemia
Trastuzumab	Breast cancer
Alemtuzumab	CLL
Bevacizumab	Colon, lung, breast cancer
Panitumumab	Colon cancer
Ranibizumab	PNH
Canakinumab	CAPS
Natalizumab	Multiple myeloma
Daclizumab	Organ transplant rejection
Gemtuzumab	Acute leukemia
Belimumab	SLE

Known/suspected Teratogens

ACE inhibitors, alcohol, aminopterin, androgens, carbamazepine, coumarins, danazol, diethyl stilbestrol, etretinate, isotretinoin, lithium, methimazole, methotrexate, phenytoin, radioactive iodine, tetracycline, trimethadione, valproate

Drugs for Osteoporosis

Inhibit bone resorption	*Promote bone formation*	*Both*
Bisphosphonates		Strontium
Calcitonin	Calcium	ranelate
Strontium		
Cinacalcet	Fluoride	
Denosumab	Teriparatide	
Gallium nitrate	Calcitriol (Vit D)	

Bisphosphonates

Less potent	Clodronate, etidronate, medronate
Potent	Alendronate, ibadronate
Most potent	Pamidronate, risedronate, tiludronate, zolendronate (5 mg yearly)

Antiepileptic Drugs		
1. Na^+ channel inactivation	2. Chloride channel opening	3. T type calcium current inhibition
Carbamazepine		
Lacosamide	Barbiturates	Ethosuximide
Lamotrigine	Benzodiazepines	Lamotrigine
Phenytoin	Gabapentin	Trimethadione
Rufinamide	Pregabalin	Valproate
Topiramate	Tiagabine	
Zonisamide	Vigabatrin	
4. k^+ channel facilitator	5. Orphan drug	6. SVA_2 inhibitor
Retigobine (ezogabine)	Felbamate	Levetiracetam

Endogenous Opioids

Proopiomelanocortins—betaendorphins, beta lipotrophins
Preproenkephalins—Met encephalin, leu encephalin

Preprodynorphins

Pure agonist—morphine, pethidine, codeine, pentazocine methadone, fentanyl, alfentanyl, remifentanyl sufentanyl

Pure antagonist—naloxone, naltrexone, nalmefene

Partial agonist–antagonist—buprenorphine

Agonist–antagonist—butorphanol, nalbuphine, pentazocine

Sufentanyl is most potent, remifentanil is shortest acting

Antidepressants

MAO inhibitors	Clorgyline, iso carboxazid, moclobamide, phenelzine tranylcypromine
Tricyclics	Amitriptyline, doxepine, imipramine, trimipramine
Tetracyclics	Amoxapine, clomipramine, dothiapine, desipramine, loxapine, nortriptyline
SSRI	Citalopram, escitalopram, fluvoxamine, fluoxetine, paroxetine, setraline

Atypical

SNRIs	Desvenlafaxine, venlafaxine, duloxetine, milnacipran
SSRE	Amineptine, tianeptine
NaSSA	Mianserin, mirtazapine
SARI	Trazodone
NADA	Bupropion
	Nefazodone is shortest acting

Tyrosine Kinase Inhibitors

Imatinib	CLL
Dasatinib	GIST
Nilotinib	ALL, MDS
Sorafenib	RCC, HCC

Erlotinib	Non-small cell lung cancer, pancreatic cancer
Gefitinib	Non-small cell lung cancer, pancreatic cancer
Vandetanib	Thyroid cancer
Ruxolitinib	Myelofibrosis
Bosutinib	CML
Ponatinib	CML
Afatinib Crizotinib Vemurafenib	NSCLC
Dabrafenib	Melanoma

Anti VEGF

Pegaptanib, pazoponib
Bevacizumab, ramucirumab, aflibercept
Axitinib, cabozatinib, lenvatinib, pazopanib

HDAC Inhibitors

Belinostat, vorinostat, romidepsin

Multikinase Inhibitors

Axitinib	RCC
Cabozatinib	Thyroid cancer
Osimertinib	NSC lung cancer
Regorafenib	Colon cancer
Vandetanib	Thyroid cancer

Insulins

Short acting	Duration of action
Aspart	2–4 hours
Glulisine	2–4 hours
Lispro	2–4 hours
Regular	3–6 hours
Inhaled	3 hours

Long acting	
NPH	10–16 hours
Detemir	12–14 hours
Glargine	20–24 hours
Degludec	up to 42 hours

Drugs of Choice for Various Conditions/Diseases

Condition/Disease	Drug of choice
Abdominal colic	Dicyclomine
Absence seizure, GTCS	Valproate
Acquired QT - prolongation	$MgSO_4$
Acute asthma (mild attack)	β_2-agonist (inhaled)
Acute asthma (severe attack)	$O_2 + \beta_2$-agonist + Corticosteroids
Acute attack of angina	Nitroglycerin (sublingual)
Acute gout	NSAIDs (except aspirin)
Acute hyperkalemia	Calcium gluconate
Acute pulmonary edema	Furosemide (loop diuretic)
Acute severe digitalis toxicity	Digibind
ADHD	Methylphenidate
Alcohol craving	Naltrexone
Alcohol withdrawal	BZDs
Alzheimer's disease	Rivastigmine/galantamine/donepezil
Anaesthetic in shock	Ketamine
Anaphylactic shock	Adrenaline (IM > SC)
Anasthetic for neurosurgery	Isoflurane
Aspirin induced asthma	Leukotriene antagonist
Atonic seizures – Myoclonic epilepsy	Valproate
Atrial fibrillation/-Atrial flutter (to maintain-sinus rhythm)	Ibutilide, flecainide

Condition/Disease	Drug of choice
Atrial fibrillation/ Atrial flutter (to control - ventricular rate)	β-blockers
Atropine poisoning	Physostigmine
AV block, sinus – bradycardia	Atropine
Benzodiazepine – poisoning	Flumazenil
Bledding esophageal varices	Terlipressin (vasopressin analogue)
Bronchodilator in COPD	Anticholinergics
Cardiogenic shock with oliguric RF	Dopamine
Cardiogenic shock	Dobutamine > dopamine
Central diabetes insipidus	Desmopressin
Cerebral edema	Mannitol
Cheese reaction	Phentolamine
Chemotherapy induced vomiting	5-HT3 antagonists (ondansetron), pethidine
Chronic asthma	Inhaled corticosteroids
Chronic cancer pain	Morphine/fentanyl
Chronic CHF	ACE inhibitors
Cirrhotic and nephrotic edema	Aldosterone antagonists (spironolactone)
CLL	Fludarabine + rituximab
Congenital QT prolongation	β-blockers
Cyanide poisoning	Nitrates
Depression, OCD	SSRIs, antidepressants
Diagnosis of myasthenia gravis	Edrophonium
Digitalis induced ventricular tachycardia	Lidocaine
Drug induced Parkinsonism	Central anticholinergics
Erectile dysfunction	Phosphodiesterase-5-inhibitors (Sildenafil)

Condition/Disease	Drug of choice
Ethylene glycol and methanol poisoning	Fomepizole
Exercise induced asthma	β_2-agonist
Familial hypercholesterolemia (Type II)	Statins
Familial combined hyperlipidemia (Type V)	Fibrates
Familial lipoprotein - lipase deficiency (Type I)	Fibrates
Familial dysbetalipoproteinemia (Type III)	Fibrates
Hypertriglyceridemia	Fibrates
Febrile seizures	Rectal diazepam
Fibrinolytic overdose	EACA
Generalized anxiety - disorders	Benzodiazepines
Heat stroke, hiccups	Chlorpromazine
Heparin induced thrombocytopenia	Direct thrombin inhibitors
Heparin overdose	Protamine sulfate
Hypertension during surgery of pheochromocytoma	Phentolamine
Hypertension in pregnancy	Methyldopa
Hypertensive emergencies in pregnancy	Hydralazine
Hypertensive emergencies	Sodium nitroprusside
Hypothyroidism	Levothyroxine
Hypovolemic shock	Intravenous crystalloids
Inducing agent for day care surgery	Propofol
Infantile spasm	Vigabatrin

Condition/Disease	Drug of choice
Inhalational agent for day care surgery	Sevoflurane, desflurane
Insomnia	BZDs
Lithium induced diabetes insipidus	Amiloride
Low tension glaucoma	Latanoprost (PG analogue)
Malignant hyperthermia	Dantrolene
Mania	Lithium
Migraine (prophylaxis)	Propranolol
Migraine (treatment)	Sumatriptan
Morning sickness	Antihistaminic (e.g. doxylamine)
Motion sickness	Scopolamine (hyoscine)
Mountain sickness	Acetazolamide
Muscle relaxant for day care	Mivacurium
Muscle relaxant for endotracheal intubation	Succinyl choline
Myasthenia gravis – cobra bite	Anticholinesterase (neostigmine)
Reversal of neuromuscular block	Anticholinesterase (neostigmine)
Mydriatic in adults	Tropicamide
Mydriatic in children	Atropine
Narcolepsy	Modafinil
Nephrogenic diabetes - insipidus	Thiazides
Nocturnal enuresis	Desmopressin
Open angle glaucoma	Beta blocker
Opioid withdrawal	Methadone
Oral anticoagulant overdose	Vitamin K
Organophosphate poisoning	Atropine

Condition/Disease	Drug of choice
Paracetamol (Acetaminophen) poisoning	N-Acetylcysteine
Partial seizure	Carbamazepine
Patent ductus arteriosus	Indomethacin
Peptic ulcer Gastroesophageal reflux disease (GERD) ZE syndrome NSAIDs induced ulcer	Proton pump inhibitors
Pheochromocytoma	Phenoxybenzamine
Postmenopausal osteoporosis Steroid induced osteoporosis	Alendronate (bisphosphonates)
Postpartum hemorrhage	Oxytocin
Postural hypotension	Midodrine
Prophylaxis of stable (classical) angina	β-blockers
Prophylaxis of variant angina	Calcium channel blockers
PSVT	Adenosine
Renovascular hypertension, hypertension with DM, gout and nephropathy	ACE inhibitors
Sedative for day care	Midazolam
Thyrotoxicosis in pregnancy	Propylthiouracil
Trigeminal neuralgia	Carbamazepine
Type 1 DM	Insulin
Type 2 DM	Metformin
Ventricular premature beat (extrasystole)	β-blockers
Vertigo	Cinnarizine
VT/VF	Lidocaine/amiodarone/procainamide

Treatment of Choice for Infections

Infection	*Drug of choice*
Actinomycosis	Penicillin G
Anaerobes	Metronidazole
Anthrax	Ciprofloxacin/doxycycline
Ascariasis (roundworm)	Albendazole
Atypical pneumonia; (mycoplasma)	Erythromycin
Babesiosis	Quinine + clindamycin
Brucella	Doxycycline + rifampin
Cholera	Doxycycline
CMV	Ganciclovir
Cryptosporidiosis	Paromomycin/nitazoxanide
Cyclosporiasis, isosporiasis	Cotrimoxazole
Diphtheria	Penicillin/erythromycin
Echinococcosis (hydatid cyst)	Albendazole
Endocarditis	Amoxicillin/clindamycin
Enterobiasis	Albendazole
Filariasis	DEC
Flukes (except fasciola)	Praziquantal
Giardiasis	Metronidazole
Gonorrhoea	Ceftriaxone
Group B streptococcus	Ampicillin
Hookworm	Albendazole
HSV	Acyclovir
Influenza A and B	Oseltamivir
Kala-azar	Liposomal amphotericin B
Legionella	Azithromycin or levofloxacin

Infection	Drug of choice
Leptospirosis	Amoxicillin
Listeria	Ampicillin + gentamicin
Lyme's disease	Doxycycline
Lymphogranuloma - venerum	Azithromycin or doxycycline
Microsporidiosis	Albendazole
MRSA	Vancomycin
Onchocerciasis (river blindness)	Ivermectin
P. falciparum	ACT (artemisinins)
P. vivax	Chloroquine
P. carinii (jiroveci)	Cotrimoxazole
Pertussis	Erythromycin
Plague	Streptomycin
Pseudomonas	Antipseudomonal β-lactam + aminoglycosides
Rheumatic fever	Benzathine penicillin
Rickettsia	Tetracyclines
Staphylococci	Penicillin
Streptococcus	Penicillin
Strongyloidosis	Ivermectin
Syphilis	Penicillin G
Tapeworm	Praziquantel
TB	INH with or without rifampicin
Toxoplasma in pregnancy	Spiramycin
Toxoplasma	Cotrimoxazole
Trichinosis	Albendazole
Trichomoniasis	Metronidazole
Trichuris	Albendazole
UTI	Cotrimoxazole
VRSA	Linezolid

Drugs of Choice for Chemoprophylaxis

Infection	*Drug of choice for chemoprophylaxis*
Bird flu	Oseltamivir
Cholera	Tetracycline
Diphtheria	Erythromycin
Gonorrhoea/syphilis	Procaine penicillin
Influenza	Amantadine
MAC	Clarithromycin/azithromycin
Malaria	Chloroquine
Meningococci	Rifampicin
P. carinii	Cotrimoxazole
Plague	Tetracycline
Rickettsia	Tetracyclines
Surgical prophylaxis	Cefazolin
Toxoplasmosis	Cotrimoxazole
Whooping cough	Erythromycin

Drugs Adverse Effects

Constipation—aluminium antacid, phenothiazines, opiates, TCA, iron, calcium, ganglion blockers

Aplastic anaemia—diclofenac, chloramphenicol, cotrimoxazole, indomethacin, phenytoin, nitrofurantoin

Tubular necrosis—aminoglycosides, amphotericin B, cisplatin, colistin, cyclosporine, sulfonamides, tetracyclines

Hypothyroidism—lithium, iodides, amiodarone, phenytoin, carbamazepine, rifampicin, methimazole, ketoconazole

Ototoxicity—aminoglycosides, chloroquine, cisplatin, aspirin, erythromycin, quinine, cisplatin, furosemide

Depression—anticonvulsant, beta blockers, barbiturates, statins, calcium channel blockers, OCP, fluoroquinolones

Asthma precipitation—NSAIDs, beta blockers, nitrofurantoin, aspirin

Seizure—betalactam antibiotics, INH, tramadol, quinolones, antipsychotics, theophylline, antidepressants

Galactorrhoea—chlorpromazine, haloperidol, metoclopramide, ranitidine, verapamil

Hepatotoxic Drugs

Hepatitis—INH, phenytoin, methyl dopa, aspirin

Hepatocellular necrosis—paracetamol

Cholestasis—OCP, androgens, anabolics, allopurinol, chlorpromazine

Granuloma—INH, sulfa, carbamazepine

Fatty change in liver—tetracycline, amiodarone, methotrexate

Hypokalemia—insulin, amphotericin B, gentamicin, penicillins, beta agonists, alfa blockers

Hyperglycemia—corticosteroids, OCP, protease inhibitors, thiazides, phenytoin, frusemide, diazoxide, thyroxine

Extrapyramidal Symptoms

Metoclopramide, OCP, TCA, haloperidol

Corticosteroid—Adverse Effects		
Osteoporosis	Growth retardation	Opportunistic infection
Cataract	Hypertension	
Glaucoma	Myopathy	
DM	Pseudotumor cerebri	
Cushingoid	Peptic ulcer	
Psychosis	Pancreatitis	

Cyclophosphamide, Side Effects

Cystitis, bone marrow aplasia, bladder cancer, pulmonary fibrosis, oncogenicity, teratogenicity, opportunistic infection

Methotrexate—Side Effects

Stomatitis
Hepatic fibrosis
Pneumonitis
Bone marrow supression
Teratogenicity
Opportunistic infection

Drugs of Choice for Protozoal Infections

Babesia	Clindamycin, quinine
B. coli	Tetracycline
Chaga's disease	Nifurtimox
Cyclospora	Cotrimoxazole
Leishmania	Sodium stibogluconate
Pneumocystis	Cotrimoxazole
Cryptosporidium	Paromomycin
Toxoplasma	Sulfadiazine + pyrimethamine
Cystode and trematode	Praziquantel
Fasciolopsiasis	Bithionol
Microfilariae	Ivermectin

Hydroxychloroquine, uses of

- Rheumatoid arthritis, palindromic rheumatism,
- Sarcoidosis, SLE, Q fever, Whipple's disease
- Porphyrea cutanea tarda, hypercalcemia
- Malaria prophylaxis, CPPD disease

Hydroxyurea, uses of

- CML, myelomonocytic leukemia
- Sickle cell anemia
- Hypereosinophilic syndrome
- Essential thrombocytosis

Praziquantel, uses of

- Intestinal flukes, neurocysticercosis, echinococcosis, diphyllobothriasis

Thalidomide, uses of

- Multiple myeloma, myelofibrosis, pheochromocytoma
- Ankylosing spondylitis, Behcet's syndrome
- Erythema nodusum leprosum, pheochromocytoma

Propranolol, uses of

- Hypertension, ataxia, tremor, portal hypertension
- Migraine prophylaxis, postcoital headache, long QT syndrome
- Hyperkalemic palsy, cocaine toxicity, portal hypertension

Minocycline, uses of

- Acne, actinomycosis, legionellosis, leprosy
- Sarcoidosis, Whipple's disease

Moxifloxacin, uses of

- Anaerobic infections, leprosy, legionellosis
- Community acquired pneumonia, MDR tuberculosis
- Plague, pelvic inflammatory disease

Metronidazole, uses of

- Amoebiasis, anaerobic infections, bacterial vaginosis
- Giardiasis, clostridial infections, *H. pylori*
- Pelvic inflammatory disease, necrotizing fasciitis
- Hepatic encephalopathy

Botulinum Toxin, uses of

- Achalasia cardia, anal fissure, dystonia, esophageal spasm
- Essential tremor, hemifacial spasm, migraine prevention
- Hyperhydrosis, tics, facial cosmesis

Albendazole, uses of

- Ascariasis, capillariasis, cutaneous larva migrans
- Cysticercosis, echinococcosis, enterobiosis, giardiasis
- Ankylostomiasis, lymphatic filariasis, loiasis.

Index

Symbols

A

B

C

M

N

O

Q

R

S

T

Reader's Notes

Reader's Notes

Reader's Notes